Listening to Children and Young People in Healthcare Consultations

ᵧy

`ᴐa

Listening to Children and Young People in Healthcare Consultations

Edited by

SARAH REDSELL

Principal Research Fellow
School of Nursing, Midwifery and Physiotherapy, University of
Nottingham

and

ADRIAN HASTINGS

General Practitioner
Senior Clinical Educator, Leicester Medical School

Foreword by
TERENCE STEPHENSON
President, Royal College of Paediatrics and Child Health

Radcliffe Publishing
Oxford • New York

Radcliffe Publishing Ltd
18 Marcham Road
Abingdon
Oxon OX14 1AA
United Kingdom

www.radcliffepublishing.com

Electronic catalogue and worldwide online ordering facility.

British Library Cataloguing in Publication Data

A catalogue record for this book is available from the British Library.

ISBN-13: 978 184619 346 0

The paper used for the text pages of this book is FSC certified. FSC (The Forest Stewardship Council) is an international network to promote responsible management of the world's forests.

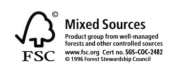

Mixed Sources
Product group from well-managed forests and other controlled sources
www.fsc.org Cert no. SGS-COC-2482
© 1996 Forest Stewardship Council

Typeset by Pindar NZ, Auckland, New Zealand
Printed and bound by TJI Digital, Padstow, Cornwall, UK

Contents

Foreword

In 2009, the Secretary of State for Health, Andy Burnham, said 'the National Health Service is a service designed by old people for old people'. He championed the view that children and young people should be involved in decisions about how health services for them are delivered and certainly there are good examples from children's hospitals around the United Kingdom and worldwide over the last two decades where children's voices have been heard in the design of emergency departments, wards and outpatient facilities.

So, this book is very timely. In November 2009, to celebrate the twentieth anniversary of the United Nations Convention on the Rights of the Child, the first reading of the Children's Rights Bill was heard in the House of Lords in the United Kingdom. In March 2010, the second reading was heard. In 2009, for the first time, the Royal College of Paediatrics and Child Health involved children and young people in the selection process for the appointment of a new Chief Executive. The College recognises that two particular groups of young people are more difficult to reach and whose voices may not be heard: adolescents and children with mental health problems. In 2009, the College launched an e-learning programme to help healthcare workers communicate better with adolescents and in 2010 we hope to undertake a similar programme of work in relation to children with mental health problems.

Listening to Children and Young People in Healthcare Consultations sets out in detail, chapter by chapter, how health professionals can best involve children in consultations and health-related decision-making. This is not icing on the cake. This is essential to successful consultations with children and young people and, in the long-term, avoids misunderstandings and ensures better care. The book provides scenarios and practical examples on how to do it. In my own continuing professional development, what I have found most useful is hearing from other expert people how they ask questions to young people about difficult and sensitive subjects. I think most of us are aware that we should ask them but many people struggle with framing the question in a way that is both empathic and informative.

Consulting with children and young people is more complicated than with adults because generally there will be three people in the room. The issues of ethics, consent and confidentiality are more complex for the same reason and are dealt with in this book. Professionals also have to learn the ability to talk in plain English to children of different developmental ages, avoiding the risk of confusing younger children and patronising older children.

If you would like to explore these difficult issues and try to improve your own practice, I commend this book to you.

Professor Terence Stephenson
President, Royal College of Paediatrics and Child Health
August 2010

About the editors

Sarah Redsell is a Principal Research Fellow in the School of Nursing, Midwifery and Physiotherapy, University of Nottingham. She is also a health visitor. Sarah's research primarily focuses on the development and evaluation of interventions to improve the health and well-being of children and young people. She has investigated the prevention of obesity during childhood, immunisation information delivery and factors affecting children's involvement in asthma consultations. She previously co-authored a book with Adrian Hastings entitled, *The Good Consultation Guide for Nurses*, which was published by Radcliffe Publishing in 2006.

Adrian Hastings is a general practitioner and senior clinical educator working for Leicester Medical School. He is course leader for the Clinical Methods Course, which teaches senior medical students a patient-centred, problem-solving approach to the consultation. The course includes instruction on the clinical assessment of children. He has led workshop courses for GPs in child health surveillance and is a visiting lecturer at De Montfort University. His research interests are in medical education with a focus on evaluating student learning of consultation skills.

About the contributors

Jo Aldridge is a senior lecturer in Social Policy and Criminology in the Department of Social Sciences at Loughborough University. She is also director of the Young Carers Research Group (YCRG), which is known internationally for its pioneering and innovative research on young carers. Jo's most recent research study was a photographic participation investigation (funded by the Economic and Social Research Council) of children who care for parents with serious mental health problems. She is currently working with Manchester Carers Forum and Child and Adolescent Mental Health Services on a project that looks at the psychological impact of caring on children and young people.

Elizabeth Anderson is a senior lecturer in the Department of Medical and Social Care Education at the University of Leicester. From a clinical career as a midwife and health visitor, Elizabeth moved to an academic career with the Department of Child Health, in Leicester, where her research interests were on sudden infant death syndrome (SIDS), poverty and deprivation. Recently she has led a regional approach to interprofessional education and published widely in this field. She is a board member of the UK Centre for the Advancement of Interprofessional Education (CAIPE). She is a National Teaching Fellow.

Heather Benjamin is a multisensory impairment consultant. She has spent 30 years teaching in special education, more specifically children with profound and multiple disabilities. For 20 years she has worked in partnership with Dorothy MacKinlay counselling profoundly disabled children and young people.

Adrian Brooke is a consultant paediatrician based in the community in Leicester, England. He is an honorary senior lecturer at the University of Leicester and contributes to the teaching of undergraduate medical students and allied health professionals at both Leicester and De Montfort universities. He has published material on respiratory and general paediatrics as well as authoring work on the healthcare of children in schools. He is the clinical lead and clinical cabinet member for children at NHS East Midlands. As a practising paediatrician he regularly undertakes specialised assessment of children referred following allegations of child abuse.

Patricia Cahill works as a general practitioner and a community paediatrician in Suffolk. She teaches communication skills to medical students as well as to established clinicians. Her research interest is communication, particularly multiparty paediatric consultations.

Cris Glazebrook is a professor of health psychology at the University of Nottingham. Her research focuses on the psychological and behavioural consequences of chronic conditions in childhood, including asthma, Tourette syndrome and HIV. Current research evaluates interventions to improve outcomes in vulnerable groups such as very premature infants and children with risk factors for obesity. She is also UK lead for a project funded by the Department for International Development which aims to encourage Zambian adolescents to participate in their healthcare. This has involved developing training programmes for health workers and educational materials for young people.

Pippa Hemingway is a lecturer in Nursing Children and Young People in the School of Nursing, Midwifery and Physiotherapy, University of Nottingham. She is a registered children's nurse. Pippa has a PhD from the Academic Division of Child Health, University of Nottingham. Her research interests primarily focus on parental perspectives regarding emergency department, urgent care and general practice attendance with sick children. Pippa is also working with ScHARR, University of Sheffield, on a project looking at consultation for childhood appendicitis.

Dorothy MacKinlay is a clinical psychologist working in hospital paediatrics at Nottingham University Hospitals NHS Trust. Her clinical interest is in working with children to give them skills to cope with challenging situations and, to this end, she has also produced a variety of preparation material aimed at empowering children to become active participants in their treatment. Her research interests are in transition from paediatric to adult services and in children's quality of life. She is the joint author of the Generic Children's Quality of Life Measure (GCQ) for children with Professor Jacqueline Collier, University of East Anglia.

Amy McPherson is a scientist in the 'Participation and Inclusion' theme at Bloorview Kids Rehab, Canada's largest children's rehabilitation hospital. She is also assistant professor at the Dalla Lana School of Public Health, University of Toronto. Amy is a health psychologist and previously taught behavioural sciences and communication skills to trainee health professionals at the University of Nottingham. Her research explores the psychological impact of long-term conditions on children and their families, and promoting children's well-being through choice and empowerment. Current research projects include how children with spina bifida participate in consultations with healthcare professionals, and the perceptions of children with disabilities around health and well-being.

Anne Willmott has been a consultant paediatrician and gastroenterologist at

Leicester Royal Infirmary since 2005. Her job involves tertiary gastroenterology, combined with acute general paediatrics and involvement in teaching and examining. She is an honorary senior lecturer at University of Leicester, and as part of her job she has been teaching medical students about consultations with children and families for several years. She also facilitates regularly on a local teaching and learning course.

Introduction

Sarah Redsell and Adrian Hastings

Children and young people present for healthcare with a range of conditions from acute through to lifelong disease, with social and psychological dimensions to the illness causing their poor health. Sometimes they encounter health professionals with specialist training, such as paediatricians, children's nurses, health visitors and school nurses. Often, however, they consult with health professionals who have more limited specialist knowledge of children, such as hospital doctors in training, general practitioners and practice nurses. Consulting with children and young people is more complicated than with adults because there are nearly always three people in the consultation (usually parent, child and health professional), and children differ in their understanding according to their cognitive ability and age. Research evidence suggests the dominant communication model in contemporary medical practice is one in which communication within a consultation takes place between a health professional and the parent as proxy for the child.[1,2] Children's contributions to consultations are limited.[2–4] and in some cases they may not participate verbally at all.[5] Where children do contribute to a consultation, it is primarily to provide information or engage with social conversation.[4–6] Health professionals rarely discuss treatment issues or provide medical information, even to older children and young people.[5]

Young people and their parents would like greater inclusion in healthcare decisions and there is systematic review evidence that children with asthma, who are involved in all aspects of their treatment, have improved clinical and psychosocial outcomes.[7,8] From a policy perspective, the National Service Framework (NSF) for Children, Young People and Maternity Services (2004) states that all health professionals must fully involve children, young people and their parents in all stages of their healthcare by 2014.[9] The purpose of this book is to raise health professionals' awareness of the need to engage with children in all aspects of the consultation, and to provide guidance on how this can be accomplished. This is achieved through a series of stand-alone chapters written by academics and health professionals in the field. The book provides the research evidence to support the involvement of children in healthcare and practical examples on how to do this during consultations with children and young people with a range of conditions. We anticipate that the book will be useful for health professionals at all stages of their career, regardless of whether their primary qualification is medical, nursing or of a profession allied to medicine.

Chapter 1 reviews the development of understanding of children's needs as recipients of healthcare. It describes how basic public health measures implemented during the Victorian era led to improvements in the length and quality of children's lives. It moves on to consider children in hospital and the restricted parental visiting policy introduced by the Victorians to prevent infection. The authors describe the work of scientists like John Bowlby and reformers such as James Robertson who sought to persuade hospitals to take account of the emotional, as well as the physical needs of sick children. This chapter guides the reader through the more recent policy and research activities that have put children at the centre of their healthcare.

The second chapter examines the literature in relation to children's development, cognition, age and communication within the consultation. The author outlines the rationale for involving children in healthcare and consultations, especially those with chronic conditions. The chapter brings together evidence identifying the factors that affect the extent of children's involvement in consultations and provides guidance for promoting their participation.

Chapter 3 describes the different dynamics within primary healthcare consultations involving a child, when varied combinations of parent(s), carer, friend and health professional can be present. The author uses vignettes to show how 'others' can be responsible for both excluding and facilitating children's contributions to a consultation, and guides health professionals towards a child-centred focus.

The fourth chapter also offers practical techniques for promoting the involvement of children in healthcare. The author describes how health professionals can make their communication with children and families more effective with subtle changes to language, body language, environment and setting. The author uses the competence framework incorporated within the Consultation Assessment and Improvement Instrument for Nurses (CAIIN) to show how communication can be improved at each stage of the consultation process.[10]

Chapter 5 explores the perspectives of different health, social and educational professionals who consult with children. Using Erikson's developmental model, the authors describe the contributions each discipline can make. They also look at interdisciplinary working in relation to children in terms of a common assessment framework, problem solving and management method.

Chapter 6 describes the experiences, often unrecognised, of children who care for their parents with chronic disease or mental illness. The author provides guidance for health professionals to heighten their awareness of the roles children often fulfil as carers of their parents. She presents the evidence for the need to support these children, who often lack advice and practical help.

The seventh chapter relates the stories of four children. Each story illustrates the concepts presented in four of the preceding chapters. It details the interactions between professionals, children and parents, and invites the reader to analyse the meanings, recognise when good communication skills have been used, and proposes alternative, more effective, responses that the professional might have made.

Chapter 8 considers the issues of consent and choice for children and young people. It examines the age of appropriate consent, parental versus child consent, 'Gillick competence', refusal of treatment and confidentiality.

The critical importance of listening to the child in relation to safeguarding procedures is described in Chapter 9. There is a description of the various types of abuse children may experience. The authors describe how failures in communication between professionals can have disastrous results for children and make suggestions for improvements based on recent serious case reviews.

Chapter 10 focuses on consulting with children with learning difficulties and other disabilities. The author describes techniques for health professionals consulting with children and young people with special needs. The chapter also explores in depth the authors' work with children with severe learning difficulties and the techniques used to communicate with them.

The last chapter explores parents' roles in preparing children who are attending the emergency department. Methods of how parents can prepare children for the encounter are discussed, along with a description of parental modelling. The chapter ends with a guide for parents that incorporates sample questions that a parent may wish to consider prior to attending a consultation, to maximise the level of their child's participation.

Throughout the book we use terms consistently. 'Professional' – qualified in health or social care – describes any person who is a trained worker interacting with children and their parents. We use the following terms for specific professions:
➤ doctor
➤ nurse
➤ therapist
➤ social worker.

When the context requires, a specific discipline label is used:
➤ paediatrician
➤ health visitor
➤ general practitioner.

The term 'parent' is used by preference, as it is nearly always the true relationship between the child and adult coming to a consultation with a professional. It encompasses biological, step- and adoptive parents. The words 'child' and 'children' are used as generic terms to encompass infants, babies, toddlers, children and young people. Words that indicate a narrower age range are used when the context requires. 'Kids' is only used in reported speech. 'Teenager' is replaced by the term 'young people', which implies that the individuals concerned are completing the transition through puberty and no longer consider themselves to be children. The term 'carer' is used as necessary when the context requires. It implies both formal care (as in a 'foster carer') and informal care roles and has the sense of the person looking after the child at the time of the consultation, with de facto responsibility for the child at that moment. More specific terms are used as appropriate to describe the relationship between child and accompanying adult (e.g. mother, father, grandmother, sister). Informal terms for carers are used in examples, case scenarios and reported speech (e.g. Mum, Dad, Gran).

REFERENCES

1 Pantell RH, Stewart TJ, Dias JK, *et al.* Physician communication with children and parents. *Pediatrics.* 1982; **70**(3): 396–402.

2 Tates K, Meeuwesen L. Doctor–parent–child communication: a (re)view of the literature. *Soc Sci Med.* 2001; **52**(6): 839–51.

3 Wissow LS, Roter D, Bauman LJ, *et al.* Patient–provider communication during the emergency department care of children with asthma. The National Cooperative Inner-City Asthma Study, National Institute of Allergy and Infectious Diseases, NIH, Bethesda, MD. *Med Care.* 1998; **36**(10): 1439–50.

4 Wassmer E, Minnaar G, Abdel Aal N, *et al.* How do paediatricians communicate with children and parents? *Acta Pædiatr.* 2004; **93**(11): 1501–6.

5 van Dulmen AM. Children's contributions to pediatric outpatient encounters. *Pediatrics.* 1998; **102**(3.1): 563–8.

6 Tates K, Meeuwesen L. 'Let mum have her say': turntaking in doctor–parent–child communication. *Patient Educ Couns.* 2000; **40**(2): 151–62.

7 Boylan P. *Children's Voices Project: feedback from children and young people about their experience and expectations of healthcare.* Commission for Health Improvement. London: DoH; 2004.

8 Guevara J, Wolf FM, Grum CM, *et al.* Effects of educational interventions for self-management of asthma in children and adolescents: systematic review and meta-analysis. *Brit Med J.* 2003; **326**(7402): 1308–9.

9 Department of Health. *The National Service Framework for Children, Young People and Maternity Services.* London: DoH; 2004.

10 Hastings AM, Redsell SA (editors). *The Good Consultation Guide for Nurses.* Oxford: Radcliffe Medical Press; 2004.

CHAPTER 1

Finding a voice: the development of children's healthcare

Sarah Redsell and Cris Glazebrook

INTRODUCTION

In this chapter we review the development of understanding of children's needs as recipients of healthcare. We begin by describing how basic public health measures implemented during the Victorian era led to improvements in the length and quality of children's lives. Then we consider children in hospital and the origins of the restricted parental visiting policy introduced by the Victorians to prevent infection. We describe the work of scientists like John Bowlby and reformers like James Robertson who sought to persuade hospitals to take account of the emotional, as well as the physical, needs of sick children. Our chapter also looks at different approaches to the care of children in hospital and explores policy changes that have allowed for greater involvement of children in healthcare.

PUBLIC HEALTH REFORM

Children's healthcare has traditionally been regarded as both protective and curative. The protective component concerns the prevention of ill health through public health measures, such as the provision of safe drinking water, sanitation and immunisation. Curative medicine relates to the treatment of particular diseases. In the UK the reforms to public health that were undertaken over 150 years ago were the first step towards increasing children's health and life expectancy.

The Industrial Revolution began towards the end of the eighteenth century. Many people moved from the countryside to the towns and cities to work in factories. In a relatively short space of time the UK economy was transformed from agricultural to industrial production.[1] Unfortunately, the existing social structures of housing, policing, education and public health lagged behind the technological advances that were being made in transport and technology.[1] The population doubled in the first 50 years of the nineteenth century from 9 million to 18 million.[2] The already existing public health problems – a lack of clean water supply, sanitation and sewage disposal – were worsened by the increased urbanisation.[2] Poor living conditions, malnutrition and ignorance (in terms of health, hygiene and medical treatment) resulted in the population being in poor health by today's standards.

Insanitary conditions had always been present in the towns and cities but they were made worse by the population acceleration.[2] People of all ages often shared rooms in damp, filthy houses and tenement buildings. There was no sanitation and only a few houses had running water. Water was usually obtained from a pump or standpipe serving several streets and only available for a few hours a day.[2] Domestic and industrial refuse and sewage were disposed of in the street and collected infrequently. Infection spread more rapidly through the urban areas and communicable diseases such as smallpox, typhus and tuberculosis were endemic. There were epidemics of cholera and scarlet fever.[3] In 1850, the death rate for children living in urban areas was much higher than for those living in rural areas.[4] Life expectancy during the mid nineteenth century was 18–25 years in the industrial areas and 40 in the countryside,[2] which is considerably shorter than the least developed countries in the world today.

High rates of poverty resulted in a poor diet both in terms of food quality and quantity. Consequently, malnutrition was commonplace among poorer children, with many suffering from rickets.[4] These malnourished children were more susceptible to the ever-present threat of infectious disease. There was a good deal of ignorance about health and hygiene in the home, as well as medical ignorance about the treatment of infectious diseases and accidental injuries. Newborn babies who could not be breast-fed were at particular risk of dying of infection introduced by the mother's dirty hands or infected cow's milk.[5] Attacks of gastro-enteritis were common and severe diarrhoea in malnourished children often led to dehydration and death. Every backyard contained refuse and sewage and became a breeding ground for flies, which carried disease into the food chain.[5] Figure 1.1 outlines the total infant mortality rates for England and Wales, 1901–99.[6] It is worth noting that during the hot summers (i.e. in 1911) the mortality rates rose due to the numbers of infants contracting diarrhoea from poorly stored food.

Children's well-being was not seen as the responsibility of the state.[4] In fact, the state took no responsibility for public services during the early Victorian era. State or charitable intervention was frowned upon and individuals were expected to take responsibility for themselves.[4] However, there was acknowledgement that something needed to be done to stop the spread of infectious disease, particularly in the industrial areas. Victorian social and administrative reformers believed that the root causes of infectious diseases needed to be tackled and initiated a widespread overhaul of water, sewage and drainage facilities.[1] Slowly legislative changes were introduced and control of public health became a matter for local and central government.[2] Eventually, water supply, sanitation and sewage disposal became the responsibility of statutory authorities.[1] These efforts gradually reduced the likelihood of disease epidemics and made a major contribution to increasing life expectancy.[1] Figure 1.1 shows the impact of these changes on infant mortality rates.[6]

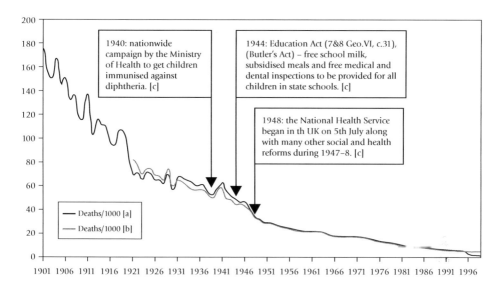

a. Source: Office for National Statistics – twentieth century mortality
b. Series DH3 No. 38 – Table 33 – Mortality statistics – Childhood, infant and perinatal. Review of the Registrar Generalon deaths in England and Wales, 2005
c. A Chronology of State Medicine, Public Health, Welfare and Related Service in Britain 1066–1999. Compiled by Michael D Warren, Faculty of Public Health Medicine of the Royal Colleges of Physicians of the United Kingdom.

FIGURE 1.1 Total infant mortality, all causes, per 1000 (infants) – England and Wales, 1901–99

The public health debate today

Public health policies are useful in providing us with an understanding of how to prevent ill health and promote good health. However, the debate about state versus individual responsibility continues. Some public health policies imply that individuals should lead a risk-free life and there are those who wish to make their own choices, which may include an element of risk. Furthermore, making a risky choice may not always be an informed decision. There are many other factors involved in an individual's decision to maintain an unhealthy behaviour. Health professionals working with children who are obese, for example, have to look beyond making recommendations to their parent(s) about a healthy diet. They may need to include an assessment of the parent's ability to understand the seriousness of the situation, an assessment of their income and their ability to provide healthy foods, together with exploring the rewards for maintaining the situation. Sometimes the gap between public health aims and individuals' lifestyle is vast.

There is now general agreement that poverty is a contributory factor in ill health. The most recent public health policy document, *Choosing Health*, emphasises the continuing need to tackle poverty and health inequalities, promote healthy living environments and healthy schools and to apply measures to help children and young people understand risky health behaviours.[7] Current public health measures include health protection interventions, such as immunisation against infectious disease; health improvement interventions to tackle individual behaviours that contribute to disease risk, such as obesity, smoking, alcohol and drugs; and patient-safety interventions to prevent healthcare institutions from harming users.

HOSPITALS AND SICK CHILDREN

Institutions that care for the sick, poor or destitute have existed since the Roman era but it was only in the eighteenth century that modern hospitals began to appear.[8] During the eighteenth century the Foundling Hospital was opened in London, which was specifically for sick and orphaned children. Once it became known that free healthcare could be obtained from the hospital sick children arrived from all over the country. Many young children and babies were abandoned at the hospital by their parents. The hospital became London's 'most fashionable charity' but it struggled to attract sufficient funds to care for the increasing numbers of children arriving at its doors.[4] Eventually it had to limit admissions to those children whose lives could actually be improved by the medical services on offer.[4]

By 1800, 35 voluntary hospitals had been founded in England and a further seven in Scotland. These were funded by wealthy benefactors who were publicly involved in their support.[4] Voluntary hospitals were mainly for the deserving poor and the destitute. The wealthy, the ordinary working-class families and those receiving poor relief from the parish were expected to pay for their own treatment at home.[4] Doctors who worked in these hospitals were largely self-supporting; often generating income by treating wealthy patients in their own homes. There were frequent disagreements between the medical staff and the hospital managers about what constituted 'destitute', with doctors unwilling to turn away deserving and interesting cases who did not fit the admission criteria.[4]

Poor sick children admitted to the voluntary hospitals were treated alongside adult patients.[8] However, mixed wards were difficult for staff to manage and there were concerns about the number of drunk and disturbed cases being admitted at night and waking the children.[4] Funds for the care of children were easier to attract when donors were certain their money would be spent only on the welfare of innocent, helpless children rather than adults suffering from what might be perceived as self-inflicted illnesses.[4] Specialist children's hospitals opened largely at the initiative of individual physicians seeking professional advancement rather than to meet a community need.[4] The mortality rates in the early children's hospitals were very high.[4] Many of the deaths were young infants and babies of destitute parents who arrived at the hospitals extremely ill and malnourished. There was often little the hospitals could do to help the large numbers of poor, sick children requiring treatment.[4]

In the UK, one of the first specialist children's hospitals was Great Ormond Street in London, which opened in 1852. The majority of its income came from its supporters through individual donations and subscriptions, a situation that remained until the formation of the National Health Service in 1948. The Admission Registers from 1852 to 1903 show the nature of children's illnesses, treatments and outcomes during that time.[3] The records suggest that children were often admitted to hospital with illnesses that were a consequence of their poverty and poor understanding about the transmission of infectious diseases. Children were treated for minor illnesses, such as catarrh and constipation, and life-threatening conditions, such as croup and rheumatic fever. Children were also admitted to the hospital with chronic diseases, such as tuberculosis, osteomyelitis and bronchiectasis. In terms of treatment, the records show that children with croup were given tracheotomies, which are rarely successful; while children with chorea were experimented on with splints, traction and sedatives.[3] The records show that doctors had their own preferences for the illnesses they treated: patients with nervous diseases are admitted by one doctor, and children with diseased joints and tubercular infections admitted by another.[3]

Lomax suggests that the most tangible measure of the condition of the children admitted to hospital was their weight.[4] Many of the children weighed so little below the modern norms that chronic malnutrition was undeniable. Lomax also points out that these children would not have displayed the liveliness present in children today and suggests that this may be why there are so few accounts of misbehaviour in the records.[4] Children in hospital were expected to adhere to stringent ward regulations and their lack of energy probably ensured they were passive recipients of healthcare.[8]

From the start, medical staff took an exploitative approach to looking after children in hospital and care revolved around the system rather than the child.[4] This approach seems to have arisen from their desire to advance medical knowledge rather than as a way of alleviating poor parents of their responsibility for their child, which was a concern at the time.[4] Poor children often remained in the hospital for at least a fortnight, irrespective of what was wrong with them.[3] The length of inpatient care was not always determined by the disease and its predicted recovery period (or remission). Children were kept in hospital for longer than necessary to provide medical staff with the opportunities for long-term clinical observation, experimental treatment of particular conditions and post-mortem examinations of those that died.[3,4] Although, in some cases, a longer stay may have been prescribed to give children respite from the domestic environment that was probably a prime factor in the development of their disease.[3] This paternalistic approach was probably essential at the time and some children clearly benefited from the nutrition, hygiene and care they received in hospital.

The enduring problem of infectious disease continued to trouble hospitals throughout England and Scotland and solutions were actively pursued. Physicians became convinced that a significant proportion of infectious disease was introduced into the wards by visitors.[4] In 1854, staff at Great Ormond Street became convinced that visitors were responsible for an outbreak of measles and scarlet fever.[4] It was decided the risk of infection could be reduced by restricting visiting times for parents. Initially this resulted in a reduction of the number of visiting days from four to two a week.[4] However, as time went on and knowledge about the spread of infectious disease increased, visiting times in most hospitals were reduced to Sunday afternoons only.

Two related traditions emerged from these early practices and became part of hospital culture for over a century. Poor sick children who were malnourished and lacking in energy were not seen to be equal in status to hospital staff. Treatment in hospital was funded by charitable donations and these children and their families were expected to be grateful. This led to an approach focused around what was best for the healthcare system (or health professionals delivering it), where the doctor 'knows best' and the child patient should be the passive recipient of care. The separation of the sick child from their family while they were in hospital, originally intended as a measure to prevent infection, became embedded in routine hospital practice. In recent years, policy makers and health professionals have sought to disentangle these customs and practices to ensure that healthcare is child- and family-focused.

CHILDREN IN HOSPITAL

The practice of separating sick children from their mothers became deeply ingrained in hospital culture and was very difficult to change.[9] However, there were some notable exceptions. As early as 1925, in Newcastle-upon-Tyne, Sir James Spence introduced the practice of allowing parents to stay in hospital with their very young children.[10] The paediatric unit in Amersham also had a long tradition of resident mothers.[11] However, the work of these innovative practitioners was not disseminated on a wider scale and the majority of children's wards continued to restrict visiting for parents. Alsop-Shields and Mohay suggest that two individuals, John Bowlby and James Robertson, played a central role in the improvement of care for children in hospital.[9]

Bowlby, in his influential report for the World Health Organization (WHO), *Maternal Care and Mental Health* (1951), claimed that children hospitalised before the age of five years were likely to have difficulty forming satisfactory relationships in adulthood and were prone to criminal or delinquent behaviour.[12] His early perspective was based on a biological model which proposes that the child's attachment to the mother is instinctual and maximises the changes of survival for the child. However, he later acknowledged that all children might not be equally vulnerable to the effects of separation from the mother during hospitalisation.[13] There has been strong criticism of health professionals' unquestioning acceptance of Bowlby's biological perspective. Hall suggests that, by focusing only on a child's biological need for their mother, health professionals ignore the social implications of the illness and the unfamiliarity of the hospital environment.[14] Hall suggests that the child has lost not only his or her mother, but also friends and other members of the family.[14] A child's reaction may also be attributed to the unfamiliar (hospital) environment with corresponding restrictions on their behaviour, illness, pain and/ or fear.[15]

James Robertson was a social worker and psychoanalyst who applied Bowlby's theory to his practice and used his political skills to change practices in children's hospitals.[9] The collaboration between Bowlby and Robertson was timely because knowledge about the spread of infection was improving, which helped to dismantle the argument that unrestricted visiting would increase infection rates.[9] The Committee on the Welfare of Children in Hospital, chaired by Sir Harry Platt, was established in 1956, 'to make a special study of the arrangements for the welfare of ill children as distinct from their medical and nursing treatment'. The Platt Report, published in 1959, made a number of recommendations for improving the care of children in hospital.[16] In particular, 'that all hospitals where children are treated will adopt the practice of unrestricted visiting, particularly for children below school age'. However, many hospitals were slow to respond. Consequently, the National Association for the Welfare of Children in Hospitals (NAWCH) (now Action for Sick Children) was formed in 1961, to raise awareness of the emotional needs of children and to encourage implementation of the Platt Report.

Bowlby remained a theorist but Robertson took a more pragmatic line.[9] His research on separation led him to develop novel techniques both to investigate the concept of 'separation' and to implement change. The stages of grief following admission to hospital and separation from the mother were captured in the film *A Two-Year-Old Goes to Hospital* (1953), which documented the experiences of Laura, hospitalised for eight days for a hernia repair at the age of two years, five months.[17] The film was shown widely for educational purposes and was instrumental in changing the attitudes of many health professionals towards the care of children in hospital.[14] In particular, it encouraged nurses to recognise that the child patient had emotional needs which were more important than hospital routines and procedures. This marked the beginning of a shift away from a health-system-centred model of care delivery towards a child- and family-centred care approach for children in hospital.

Despite a good deal of evidence that separating children from their parents in hospital may have adverse effects it took a long time for the majority of children's wards to implement unrestricted visiting for parents. Following the Platt Report changes emerged gradually beginning with a relaxation of daytime visiting hours moving towards unrestricted visiting for parents. In 1975, NAWCH carried out a survey of 800 wards and found that only 20% had unrestricted visiting, 33% allowed daytime visiting but the remainder only allowed visiting after lunch. Thirty years after the Platt Report, one study found that although a few wards had unrestricted visiting for parents, others were restrictive and discouraging in their practices.[18] Another study conducted in Dublin in 1989 found that the number of overnight resident parents in the National Children's Hospital was 38.9%.[19] This study also found that children with a resident parent were likely to spend fewer days in hospital with a mean length of stay of 2.88 days compared with children with non-resident parents who had a mean length of 4.16 days. Today children's wards are usually open all hours to parents/carers, although there are still restricted visiting hours for other visitors.[9]

Although relaxing the rules about visiting hours was seen as a vital step towards acknowledging children's and families' emotional needs, improvements to the actual care of children while in hospital was also required. Early work identified the negative effects of long-term hospital care or 'hospitalisation' on the health of infants and children.[20] Levy explored the traumatic effects of surgery and suggested that adverse outcomes could be improved if: a) children were provided with a truthful explanation of what would happen; b) the mother was present before and after surgery; and c) adequate sedation was given to the child.[21,22] The Platt Report identified that going into hospital might be traumatic for a child and recommended appropriate preparation. 'The risk that any child will be disturbed by hospital admission can be reduced by suitable preparation of both parents and children'.[16] In 1967, the NAWCH published *Coming into Hospital*, a booklet to help parents prepare children for the experience of hospital care.[23] Providing information specifically for children about hospital care was another important milestone in recognising that their needs went beyond catering for their physical well-being.

In the intervening years, there have been a number of policy developments that have led to changes to the care of children in hospital. The UK government's White Paper The Welfare of Children and Young People in Hospital was published in 1993.[24] It advocated that specially qualified professionals should meet children's health needs and that staff training in the developmental and emotional needs of children is essential to a high-quality service. *The Patient's Charter: services for children and young people* followed in 1996 and reflected the common belief that their parents are able to represent their children's views.[25] In 1997, the House of Commons' Health Committee further examined the specific health needs of children and young people and called for full explanation of proposed treatment at an appropriate level for the child's age.[26]

BOX 1.1 Elements of family-centred care[27,28]

- Recognising the family as a constant in the child's life.
- Facilitating parent–professional collaboration at all levels of healthcare.
- Honouring the racial, ethnic, cultural and socio-economic diversity of families.
- Recognising family strengths and individuality and respecting different methods of coping.
- Sharing complete and unbiased information with families on a continual basis.
- Encouraging and facilitating family-to-family support and networking.
- Responding to child and family development needs as part of healthcare practices.
- Adopting policies and practices that provide families with emotional and financial support.
- Designing healthcare that is flexible, culturally competent and responsive to family needs.

In the early 1990s, the family-centred approach to paediatric healthcare was developed in the US. The family-centred approach encourages health professionals to shift away from traditional approaches to health service delivery to the involvement of families in all aspects of the planning, delivery and evaluation of healthcare. Box 1.1 outlines the nine elements of family-centred care.[27,28] Implementation of the family-centred approach has been variable in the UK and, although the majority of children's wards adopt some of the features, gaps still remain, which can lead to communication difficulties between parents and health professionals.[29] The family-centred approach is still viewed as 'best practice' but there is currently insufficient evidence of its effectiveness when compared with standard or professional-led care.[29]

In 1999, Action for Sick Children launched the Millennium Charter outlining ten standards for the care of sick children in hospital (*see* Box 1.2).[30] These have now been incorporated by the European Association for Children in Hospital (EACH), which is the umbrella organisation for member associations involved in the welfare of all children, before, during and after a hospital stay.

BOX 1.2 Action for Sick Children (1999) Millennium Charter[30]

- All children shall have equal access to the best clinical care within a network of services that collaborate with each other.
- Health services for children and young people should be provided in a child-centred environment separately from adults so that they are made to feel welcome, safe and secure at all times.
- Parents should be empowered to participate in decisions regarding the treatment and care of their child through a process of clear communication and adequate support.
- Children should be informed and involved to an extent appropriate to their development and understanding.
- Children should be cared for at home with the support and practical assistance of community children's nursing services, unless the care that they require can only be provided in hospital.
- All staff caring for children shall be specifically trained to understand and respond to their clinical, emotional, developmental and cultural needs.
- Every hospital admitting children should provide overnight accommodation for parents, free of charge.
- Parents should be encouraged and supported to participate in the care of their child when they are sick.
- Every child in hospital shall have full opportunity for play, recreation and education.
- Adolescents will be recognised as having different needs to those of younger children and adults. Health services should therefore be readily available to meet their particular needs.

Information for children coming into hospital: research findings

A number of research studies were conducted during the latter part of the twentieth century exploring the effects of hospitalisation on the child, for example Taylor and

Connor.[19] It is now difficult to interpret the evidence from this research because the care of children in hospital has changed beyond recognition and what was appropriate care in the 1970s and 1980s is not appropriate now. Furthermore, children's status has improved since the 1950s. There is general agreement that hospitalisation can be stressful for both the child and parents.[31] There is evidence that preparation for surgery and increased parental presence, while in hospital, can reduce a child's anxiety.[32] There is also evidence that parents benefit from additional support and this is reflected in the improved recovery and psychological adjustment of their children.[32]

The practice of providing children with information about going into hospital, surgery and invasive procedures has now been established. However, there have been criticisms that many of the surgical preparation leaflets are directed at parents rather than children.[31] Smith and Callery suggest that children age 7–11 can identify their own information needs and should be actively involved in the development of their own pre-admission education.[31] However, the design of both the format and content of much of the information has been led by health professionals. This has inevitably resulted in information that health professionals think children need to know rather than what they may actually need to know. Often this information does not take account of a child's age and cognitive ability and the readability of the text is sometimes inappropriate.[33] Clearly hospital-based care has made great progress in the understanding and delivery of care to children but some gaps remain. More child involvement is needed in both the design and content of health information.

INVOLVING CHILDREN IN HEALTHCARE

There have now been several government policy documents and legislative acts which emphasise the importance of children and young people growing up in a healthy environment. *Every Child Matters: change for children* sets out the national framework for local change programmes to build services around children and young people.[34] This document emphasises maximising opportunity and minimising risk. It envisions refocusing core services from dealing with the consequences of difficult children's lives to preventing those difficulties that cause children's lives to go wrong in the first place. This includes, for example, the need to provide funding for additional nursery places and the need to identify those children at risk of social exclusion at a sufficiently early stage, so intervention can be put in place to ensure they reach their potential. The document also emphasises the need to consult with children and young people at all stages of service redesign.[34]

There is also increasing emphasis on providing patients with information and choice about health services, which includes children and their families.[35,36] In 2004, the National Service Framework for Children, Young People and Maternity Services was launched.[37] The core standards emphasise the need for health services to target children from disadvantaged backgrounds from pre-natal care, throughout childhood and across the transition into early adult life. Both the need for ongoing staff training and development, to keep pace with changes in children's understanding of healthcare issues, and the need for changes in service provision run through the document. Standard 3 covers professionals directly communicating with children and young people. It explicitly states that the views of children, young people and families must be valued when planning, delivering and evaluating services. It also states that 'health professionals must be fully involving children in healthcare decisions by 2014'.[37]

Research reporting children's perspectives on communication with UK primary care health professionals is not available. However, there is some research reporting primary care health professionals' views of consulting with children. A recent survey of general practitioners and practice nurses who manage children with asthma found that health professionals have mixed approaches to involving children in their consultations.[38] These range from empowerment to a more didactic approach, with most respondents reporting that they found achieving concordance with children difficult.

Primary care health professionals such as general practitioners and practice nurses are frequently consulted by children or young people and their parents.[39] To prepare the healthcare professional for this, all undergraduate courses in medicine/nursing include child health teaching, both theoretically and clinically. However, in hospital, the ratio of registered paediatric nurses to unqualified staff working on a hospital ward is 70:3037.[40] The numbers of practitioners working in primary care with additional paediatric training has not been documented. However, it seems likely that many practitioners do not have specialist qualifications in paediatrics. Considering the time that may have elapsed since their basic training, and the changing dynamics of paediatric healthcare, some generalist practitioners may need updating in relation to involving children in their consultations.

Many children and young people want greater involvement in their own healthcare and there is evidence that participating in consultations improves children's understanding of their illness.[41] The General Medical Council (GMC) have produced helpful guidance for practitioners who work with children that suggests they should 'involve children and young people in discussions about their care'.[42] 'Involvement' is likely to range from informed assent, which might be appropriate for young children, through to active participation in all aspects of the consultation (including assessment, problem solving and decision-making), which might be appropriate for young people. However, age may not be the only determining factor when it comes to assessing the extent to which children wish to be involved in a consultation.[38] Health professionals will also need to be able to assess a child's cognitive ability to determine the approach needed.[38] Some children may wish to be passive participants in their own healthcare and professionals will need special skills to ensure that this is actually their wish and not a response to lack of understanding about what is being asked or offered. Clearly, there is work to be done to ensure that health professionals understand and implement both the research findings and policy agenda for children's involvement in healthcare.

CONCLUSION

Children's healthcare has come a long way in the past 150 years. Preventative and curative interventions to improve children's health and quality of life have continued to develop. In this chapter we have discussed the origins of health professionals' views of healthcare for children. The development of medical paternalism during the Victorian era resulted in an overemphasis on physical care of the passive child patient. However, the extent to which children can be actively involved in decisions about their health is still being debated among policy makers, professional groups and the research community today. The acknowledgement of children as active participants within healthcare consultations will be slow to implement. However, health professionals are beginning to consult directly with children of all ages; to communicate with them about all aspects of their healthcare and to involve them in decision-making about treatment options.

REFERENCES

 1 McLean D (editor). *Public Health and Politics in the Age of Reform: cholera, the state and the Royal Navy in Victorian Britain*. London: IB Tauris; 2005.
 2 Hodgkinson R (editor). *Public Health in the Victorian Age*. Farnborough, Hants, England: Gregg International Publishers; 1973.
 3 Tanner A. Victorian children on the wards. *Lancet*. 2002; **359**(9309): 897–8.
 4 Lomax EM. Small and special: the development of hospitals for children in Victorian Britain. *Med Hist Suppl*. 1996; (16): 1–217.
 5 Littler W (editor). *Recollection and Reflections: Victorian childhood*. Coventry, England: Rennison Publications; 1997.
 6 Child Health Safety Website. England and Wales Total Infant Mortality 1901 to 1999 [Graph]. In: Vaccines did not save us: two centuries of official statistics. Available at: http://child healthsafety.wordpress.com/graphs/ (accessed 20 May 2010).
 7 Department of Health. *Choosing Health: making healthier choices easier*. London: The Stationery Office; 2004.
 8 Levene A, Reinarz J, Thornton S, Williams A. Who let them in? Eighteenth century hospital care for children in England and Scotland: a preliminary enquiry. *Arch Dis Child*. 2007; **92**(Suppl. 1): A67.
 9 Alsop-Shields L, Mohay H. John Bowlby and James Robertson: theorists, scientists and crusaders for improvements in the care of children in hospital. *J Adv Nurs*. 2001; **35**(1): 50–8.
10 Spence J. The care of children in hospital. *Brit Med J*. 1947; **1**: 125–30.
11 MacCarthy D, Lindsay M, Morris I. Children in hospital with mothers. *Lancet*. 1962; **282**(24): 603–8.
12 Bowlby J (editor). *Maternal Care and Mental Health*. Geneva: World Health Organization; 1951.
13 Bowlby J (editor). *Attachment*. Harmsworth: Penguin; 1971.
14 Hall D. Social and psychological care before and during hospitalisation. *Soc Sci Med*. 1987; **25**(6): 721–32.

15 Charles C, Gafni A, Whelan T. Shared decision-making in the medical encounter: what does it mean? (or it takes at least two to tango). *Soc Sci Med.* 1997; **44**(5): 681–92.

16 Platt H. *The Welfare of Children in Hospital.* London: HMSO; 1959.

17 Robertson J. *A Two-Year-Old Goes to Hospital.* New York: New York University Film Library; 1953.

18 Thornes R. *Where Are the Children?* London: Caring for Children in the Health Services Consortium; 1987.

19 Taylor MR, O'Connor P. Resident parents and shorter hospital stay. *Arch Dis Child.* 1989; **64**(2): 274–6.

20 Spitz R (editor). *Hospitalisation: an enquiry into the genesis of psychiatric conditions in early childhood.* New York: International Universities Press; 1945.

21 Levy D. Child patients may suffer psychic trauma after surgery. *Mod Hosp.* 1945; **65**: 51–2.

22 Levy DM. Psychic trauma of operations in children. *Am J Dis Child.* 1945; **69**: 7–25.

23 Action for Sick Children. *Coming into Hospital.* Stockport, England: Action for Sick Children (previously National Association for the Welfare of Children in Hospital); 1967.

24 Department of Health. *The Welfare of Children and Young People in Hospital.* London: The Stationery Office; 1993.

25 Department of Health. *The Patient's Charter: services for children and young people.* London: The Stationery Office; 1996.

26 Department of Health. *The Specific Health Needs of Children and Young People: second report of the House of Commons Health Select Committee.* London: The Stationery Office; 1997.

27 Trivette CM, Dunst CJ, Allen S, Wall L. Family-centredness of the *Children's Health Care Journal. Child Health Care.* 1993; **22**(4): 241–56.

28 Johnson BH. The changing role of families in health care. *Child Health Care.* 1990; **19**: 234–41.

29 Shields L, Pratt J, Davis L, Hunter J. Family-centred care for children in hospital. *Cochrane Database of Systematic Reviews 2007.* Issue 1. Art. No.: CD004811. DOI: 10.1002/14651858. CD004811.pub2.

30 Action for Sick Children. The Millennium Charter for children's health services. *Cascade.* 1999; **32**(Sep): 12.

31 Smith L, Callery P. Children's accounts of their preoperative information needs. [See comment]. *J Clin Nurs.* 2005; **14**(2): 230–8.

32 Walder C (now Glazebrook C). Psychological aspects of day-case surgery for children. University of Nottingham; PhD thesis 1992.

33 Redsell S. A study examining the psychosocial characteristics of bedwetting children and the impact of a multimedia program and written information on treatment outcomes. University of Nottingham; PhD thesis 2000.

34 HM Government. *Every Child Matters: change for children.* London: Department for Education and Skills; 2004.

35 Department of Health. *Building on the Best: choice, responsiveness and equity in the NHS.* London: The Stationery Office; 2003.

36 Department of Health. *Better Information, Better Choice, Better Health.* London: DH Publications; 2004.

37 Department of Health. *Core Standards: National Service Framework for Children, Young People and Maternity Services*. London: DH Publications; 2004.

38 McPherson A, Redsell S. Factors affecting children's involvement in asthma consultations: a questionnaire survey of general practitioners and primary care asthma nurses. *Prim Care Respir J*. 2009; **18**(1): 15–20.

39 Rowlands S, Moser K. Consultation rates from the general practice research database. *Brit J Gen Pract*. 2002; **52**(481): 658–60.

40 Smith F. *PNAE Staffing Survey Findings*. London: Royal College of Nursing; 2007. Available at: www.rcn.org.uk/__data/assets/powerpoint_doc/0016/111562/PNAE_staffing_survey_findings.ppt (accessed 20 May 2010).

41 Boylan P. *Children's Voices Project*. London: Commission for Health Improvement; 2004.

42 General Medical Council (GMC). *0–18 Years: guidance for all doctors*. London: GMC; 2007. Available at: www.gmc-uk.org/static/documents/content/GMC_0-18_0911.pdf (accessed 20 May 2010).

CHAPTER 2

Involving children: why it matters

Amy McPherson

INTRODUCTION

Many health professionals understand the importance of providing information to adult patients and involving them in decision-making about their treatment. However, the involvement of children and young people in their own healthcare has been altogether more contentious. As outlined in the first chapter, it has been recognised only relatively recently that children have multifaceted needs in a health context. Yet, despite significant improvements in children's services, it would appear that not all health professionals routinely involve children in their healthcare generally, or in healthcare consultations specifically.[1]

This chapter outlines the rationale for involving children in healthcare and consultations, especially children with chronic conditions. It also brings together evidence identifying factors which affect the extent of children's involvement in consultations and guidelines for promoting their participation. For ease, the term 'children' refers to children and young people in this chapter.

WHAT DO WE MEAN BY INVOLVEMENT?

Participation, shared decision-making, partnership, inclusion – all these terms are used by different authors when discussing the involvement of children in healthcare. Others talk about trust, respect, choice and truth as essential components of interactions with children. Clearly, there is no one way of defining 'involvement' of children in healthcare, in the same way that literature around adult's involvement in health-related decision-making and informed choice has struggled to come up with a universal concept.[2] As with adults it is likely that there are different 'levels' of involvement, or a continuum. One end of the continuum can be old-fashioned paternalism or complete dependence upon a medical professional, with absolute autonomy at the other. It is unlikely, and mostly inappropriate that a child would be master of their own health-related destiny, making decisions in a vacuum without support or input from medical professionals and other adults. Children differ in their need for autonomy; some want to decide their treatment for themselves, some want their doctor to decide for them, while others wish to share the choices with their doctor and feel part of the decision-making process.[3] This suggests that health professionals need to take such individual differences into account, rather than make assumptions regarding their desire (or lack of) to be involved in health-related decisions. However, it appears that many health professionals struggle to establish the child's preference of where they wish to sit on the continuum at any one time. This is not confined to child populations; research on the support needs of parents making health-related decisions for their children revealed that parents wished to choose their own level of participation and that they expected health professionals to ascertain their preference.[2] Therefore, health professionals working with children should aim to establish their preferred level of involvement and work with them to facilitate their participation where desired.

WHY IS IT IMPORTANT TO INVOLVE CHILDREN IN THEIR HEALTH?

There are many strands to the argument for involving children in their health. All children must engage in certain health behaviours as they grow and develop. Cleaning teeth, controlling bladder and bowels, and eating a range of foods all require the child's involvement to be successful. However, a lifespan view can also be taken. Evidence has shown that attitudes towards health behaviour in adulthood are often rooted in early experiences, suggesting that it is important for positive health behaviours to start in the early years.[4] Health policy in the UK and many other countries puts the responsibility for health squarely upon the individual, illustrated by health promotion campaigns such as eating '5 a Day', alcohol awareness and increasing physical activity.[5-7] Therefore, if adults are expected to be responsible for their own health, it seems implausible that this can occur without any form of preparation earlier in life. Indeed, being actively involved in healthcare decisions from an early age may foster a sense of control or confidence in performing specific health-related skills, termed self-efficacy.[8] A belief in our ability to influence things is connected with good emotional health and together with the opportunity to make our own decisions, this helps to build self-confidence and emotional resilience.[9] Bury and colleagues reinforce this, in their view to become competent adult decision makers, children must have had experience of making decisions, even if they make mistakes.[10] Parental behaviour is also crucial, as modelling is a powerful method of learning how to act in different situations.[11,12] Thus, the behaviour of a parent in consultations may impact upon a child's later participation in health interactions.

In order to provide child-centred healthcare, professionals must have an awareness of their own behaviour in interactions with children and their families, as this may have a direct impact upon children's future compliance.[13] Communication during consultations is likely to play a key role in building relationships between health professionals, children and their parents. Actions such as asking for opinions, checking understanding and negotiating treatment plans all facilitate partnership building.[14] Furthermore, children can provide important information to help the clinician assess the severity and impact of symptoms and plan future care.[14]

This ethos is emphasised in the recent National Service Framework for Children, Young People and Maternity Services, which explicitly states that 'Healthcare professionals need to communicate directly with children and young people, by listening to them and attempting to see the world through their eyes' (Standard 3, p. 87) and goes on to say that 'health professionals must be fully involving children, young people and their parents in all stages of their healthcare by 2014'.[15] This policy document reflects calls from children to be more involved in their healthcare. The Children's Voices Project compiled feedback directly from children and young people on a range of health services, taken from 59 separate reports from voluntary organisations and statutory agencies in the UK.[16] The report for the Commission for Health Improvement highlighted that a considerable number of children are unhappy at the lack of their inclusion in healthcare and want more information and involvement in decision-making; one child revealed that, 'You do get a say, but basically they ignore it – that's not right' (p. 25).[16] Parents of children with asthma agree that health professionals should communicate directly with their children and listen to their concerns, while also addressing parental worries.[17]

Instead, many clinicians still rely on parents' assessment of symptoms to guide diagnosis and treatment, despite research suggesting that parents and children often give conflicting reports of functioning and that even very young children are capable of observing and assessing their own symptoms.[18,19] The provision of healthcare information can confer psychological benefits for children facing hospitalisation or other major procedures in terms of reduced levels of fear and distress.[20] Furthermore, evidence suggests that socialising children into participating in their own healthcare can promote confidence and self-control, which can lead to improvements in both psychological and clinical outcomes.[21–23] Conversely, the passivity of children in consultations is unlikely to produce feelings of self-control and confidence, let alone the specific skills required to make appropriate health-related decisions throughout childhood and adulthood.

WHY IS IT PARTICULARLY IMPORTANT TO INCLUDE THOSE WITH CHRONIC ILLNESSES?

Children with chronic illnesses face ongoing visits to healthcare professionals at outpatient clinics or in primary care, sometimes for several years or even a lifetime. Conditions such as asthma and diabetes rely on patients using self-management techniques, whereby they monitor their symptoms and respond according to a predetermined plan. When children are very young, parents are usually responsible for following the plan, ensuring medications are taken correctly and behavioural aspects of the plan are adhered to (e.g. avoiding known asthma triggers). As children get older, however, they must take on the responsibility of managing their own condition, so it is vital they have both the skills and the confidence to make appropriate decisions.[24] A recent systematic review reflected a substantial body of work when it found that those children with asthma who are involved in their treatment and learn the necessary skills, feel in control of their condition and have better outcomes, including improved lung function, reduced school absence and restricted activity, improved self-efficacy and lower use of emergency services.[25] Furthermore, childhood chronic conditions can impact upon psychosocial well-being in adulthood if appropriate coping strategies are not adopted.[26] Therefore, failure to involve children with chronic conditions in their healthcare can result not only in sub-optimal management in childhood, but also has serious ramifications for health later in life.

There are anxieties that children are incapable of making the complex decisions required for effectively managing a chronic condition. However, it has been shown that children *do* have the ability to make healthcare decisions and that these abilities can be enhanced through education. A series of studies in the 1980s and early 1990s showed how training children in health-related decision-making reduced stress stemming from perceived vulnerability to illness.[23,27,28] The researchers encouraged children to consider the context of their symptoms (e.g. possible causal factors, similar symptoms experienced in the past, potential courses of action) before seeking input from a health professional. These studies demonstrated not only the competence of children to integrate information and beliefs, but also an ability to communicate effectively with professionals when given unhurried and non-judgemental conditions. Conversely, if information is withheld from children, they may conclude that they lack the ability to understand medical information and therefore have no motivation for seeking health-related information in the future.[12]

The clinician, however, still plays a key role in the management of a child's condition: the Asthma Exemplar in the National Service Framework for Children, Young People and Maternity Services demonstrates that, in order for the child to have well-managed asthma, the clinician should enter into a care partnership with the child and their family, which involves negotiating an agreed plan for the child's care.[15] It is improbable that a child's condition can be best managed without the active engagement of the child and it is unlikely that a child will be actively engaged without being fully involved in medical consultations.

FACTORS AFFECTING CHILDREN'S INVOLVEMENT IN CONSULTATIONS

There is mixed evidence around the factors that affect the participation of children in consultations. The observational work that has been undertaken, for example by Tates and others, reported extremely low levels of child involvement, and in some cases no involvement at all.[14,29–31] This work, along with more qualitative enquiries, suggests that the extent of a child's involvement in their consultation depends on a wide variety of factors associated with the key people involved, namely the child, parent(s) and health professional. The physical environment and organisational ethos can also impact upon the involvement of the child in healthcare consultations.

Child factors

Age and cognitive ability

The impact of age on involvement has been investigated, although no consistent pattern has emerged and it is difficult to draw conclusions as existing studies use varying age ranges. Generally, older children tend to demonstrate more active involvement than younger children.[30,32] In a recent survey of primary care doctors and nurses, age was ranked as the second most important factor (after cognitive ability) affecting the involvement of children in consultations.[33] The respondents' written comments revealed differing approaches to involvement, with some feeling that it was 'more appropriate' in older children, while others reported involving children from a much younger age. However, ability and willingness to participate in healthcare is not necessarily age-related; when discussing insulin injections with children with diabetes, Alderson and colleagues found that some children aged four reported happily injecting themselves, whereas others aged 11 still wanted their mothers to inject them.[34] More conventionally, other studies have found that children under 10 view a partnership with the health professional as less important than children aged 10–12.[35] Researchers have set the age a little lower, arguing that children of primary school age (from six onwards) can be both interested and able to participate in their consultations.[36] However, they caution that assumptions should not be made that every child in this age range is going to want, or be ready, to participate in their primary care consultation. In situations where a series of consultations take place, for example in managing chronic conditions, it is often necessary for the consultation style to evolve over time; so where the consultations may be dyadic (between the health professional and parent) initially, they become more triadic (adding the child into the relationship) over time. This does not just refer to the child getting older, but also reflects the trust and rapport that should develop over multiple consultations.

Of course, bound up with the age of the child is their cognitive ability, which health professionals have reported as being the most influential factor in the decision to involve a child in their consultation in the aforementioned survey, reflecting a belief that understanding, maturity and language can vary in children of the same age.[33] While undoubtedly true, this can also be problematic as health professionals often assume children's ability to understand complicated concepts of health and illness to be lower than it is in reality.[29] Work in the 1980s focused upon a Piagetian stage model for children's understanding of health and argued that children's concepts of illness are determined and constrained by their stage of cognitive development.[37] The stages represent the progress of cognitive development, charting the ability to understand the concepts of self and others, internal versus external and cause and effect. Bee and Boyd provide a good summary in *The Developing Child*.[11]

However, since that work, there have been numerous examples of children understanding more than their 'stage' of development would predict, such as children as young as five years old differentiating between a physical illness (chicken pox) and a psychological one (depression).[38] Given this evidence, including the work of Alderson *et al.*, it is clear that decisions on involvement cannot be based solely upon age-related cognitive ability, as some children are clearly in advance of child development theories about what they 'should' be able to understand given their chronological age.

A more useful concept is that of 'scaffolding', whereby children can be helped to extend beyond their current level of comprehension.[39] By taking into account the child's current grasp of a particular issue and providing contingent support, adults act as coaches to assist children in achieving a level of understanding that they would be unable to reach alone.[40,41] A practical example of this is teaching a child with asthma how to use a Metered-Dose Inhaler (MDI) with a spacer. Using an MDI requires a number of steps, which must be followed to ensure that the medication is delivered effectively. To teach a child how to do this a health professional may first demonstrate the procedure themselves, talking through each step. They may then demonstrate it again, but this time involve the child, for example by asking them to shake the inhaler before each puff or count to ten out loud while the professional inhales. The next time, the child can demonstrate the procedure, either themselves or on a teddy (for younger children), while the health professional provides reminders if necessary. As the task becomes more familiar to the child, the professional withdraws their support further until the child can perform the task on their own. For some children, this process may happen over multiple consultations. For very young children, it will also be important for the parents to have a clear understanding of the process. However, the child can still be involved; most toddlers can shake an inhaler, even if the parent has to do it correctly before actually administering it.

Of course, when considering the level of a child's understanding, the health professional needs to consider what they are asking the child to do. Simply engaging them in social talk or asking them to report when they feel pain during a physical examination will not demand much complex thinking from a child. However, asking them to recall a medication regime or consider possibilities, for example when weighing up treatment options, may only be appropriate for those with greater cognitive abilities and experience, or where a child can be helped to develop beyond their current level of understanding.

Experience and illness characteristics

Professionals may find it helpful to consider the experience of the child, including their history of health and illness, their diagnosis and the seriousness of the situation. A health professional may assume that a child who has lived with a condition for a while does not need as much involvement in a consultation as one who is newly diagnosed, and may not want to risk offending a child and their family by repeating basic information.[33] Yet, this assumption may well be erroneous; research in a paediatric respiratory clinic demonstrated that the length of time since a diagnosis of asthma was unrelated to asthma knowledge.[22] Therefore, education should be reinforced for children and young people regardless of how long they have had their condition, which ideally includes active involvement of children in their own care. Involving them in their consultations is an ideal way of communicating that the health professional considers them capable of looking after their health, that they have an important role in their healthcare and that their views will be considered. A child's experiences of health professionals and healthcare environments may have a lasting effect on them well into adulthood, and negative experiences may prevent them from seeking care or raising their views with health professionals in the future. Coyne has written about factors which hinder children's involvement in consultations, even when they actively seek participation, including: not being listened to, fear of causing 'trouble' by asking questions, feeling unwell, not having enough time with the health professionals, being disbelieved, not being able to contact health professionals and being ignored.[1,42] It is not hard to see that if children experience interactions with these characteristics there are likely to be negative consequences for future healthcare interactions, both in childhood and as adults.

When a condition is life-threatening, child patients and their parents may prefer a more paternalistic approach. However, in chronic or ongoing conditions building a partnership between health professional and the child is more desirable.[10] Researchers have found varying levels of involvement in children with different conditions. For example, in Angst and Deatrick's study, children with cystic fibrosis did not have input into planning their future care, even when they expressed a wish for involvement, yet children with scoliosis reported having the opportunity to make decisions over operations and participate in joint discussions.[43]

It may also be that children do not consider themselves to be unwell or requiring treatment, which can be a considerable challenge to health professionals. In conditions such as bed-wetting or constipation and soiling, the family may have normalised the behaviour in order to reduce the stigma upon the child, so that the child may not perceive it to be something which requires great engagement from them, either in the consultation or in subsequent attempts to treat the condition. Working with the child and family to identify how salient the condition is to all members of the family is crucial in order for treatment or management to be successful.[10]

Willingness and individual characteristics

Even if a child is cognitively able to discuss their condition with a health professional, they may not actually *want* to participate and that should be respected. Even when health professionals make repeated efforts to involve children, some will still not respond, either due to their general temperament, or their mood on that particular day.[35] As discussed above, children may have been socialised into a very passive consultation style, which affects their responsiveness to a health professional's attempts at engagement. Particular activities may be especially problematic; for example, children's responses may dwindle if they feel that they are being 'tested', so the health professional must be sensitive to this when assessing their knowledge or competence.[44] Some children's preference may be for communication to be between their parent and the health professional and for their parent to explain it to them afterwards. The child may want to actively participate on some occasions and have their parent negotiate with the health professional on their behalf on other occasions. However, this still reflects the child exercising choice and sometimes the child's only way of exerting choice is to withdraw.[10] It may take time for children to build a rapport with the health professional and feel sufficiently confident to contribute to discussions, so repeated opportunities must be provided to enable the child to contribute in their own time. Of utmost importance is that children are offered the chance to participate if they so wish and that the choice is not taken away from them by the adult participants in the consultation.

Summary of child factors: some useful questions to consider
➤ What am I asking the child to do?
➤ How long have they been unwell?
➤ What experience of healthcare settings have they had?
➤ How well does the child know the health professionals?
➤ What other developmental tasks have they mastered?
➤ How willing are they to be involved?
➤ What are the child's priorities, both during and outside of the consultation?

Parental factors
Unsurprisingly, parents play a key role in consultations with their child and a health professional. From the start, it is unlikely that the child would be seeing a health professional without the involvement of the parent. Parents are 'gatekeepers', both to accessing health professionals and also to information on diagnosis, treatments and so on. Parents can be vital to the management of a child's chronic condition, both positively, through encouraging compliance, and negatively, through lack of support and understanding. Parental behaviour also highlights the child's role further as '[i]f parents are irresponsible then the child's role is even more important'.[33]

Along with the health professional, parents are also largely responsible for the extent the child is included in a consultation, as their behaviour can both exclude children from the discussion and facilitate their participation. If a parent is supportive of a child's involvement, the child is more likely to participate.[45] Equally, parents can be effective in shutting down any child involvement in the consultation by talking over the child, answering health professionals' questions or, more explicitly, by asking the child to leave the room or discussing treatment options at a later date on the telephone.[29,35] The body of work by Tates and colleagues has demonstrated that parents are powerful agents in determining whether a child is included in the consultation. In their study of primary care consultations, they report that parents often treat their child as absent even when health professionals attempt to engage with the child in a consultation. This can be pervasive, as Tates *et al.* report that, 'Frequently, the GPs accept this parental role of speaking for their child, shift their alignment and co-construct a dyadic interaction with the parent, which renders the child as a non-addressed participant'.[46]

Parents often have significant information needs themselves during a consultation and they may express these by taking a proactive role during the consultation. This may then leave less opportunity for their child's active involvement. When asked to comment upon the child's need to be involved in a consultation, a paediatrician in Garth *et al.*'s study described her view that 'the parent's needs often tend to overwhelm it'.[35] Parents and children also tend to differ in their primary concerns about illness. In cases of serious illness, the parent is likely to be understandably highly anxious and, indeed, parents report information about the prognosis of the disease to be their chief concern, while most children and adolescents rate information about personal or bodily concerns to be most important.[47] Similarly, children with asthma often worry about the embarrassment of taking their medications in front of friends, while parental anxieties are more likely to stem from the potential effects of steroids on the child's physical growth.[4,48] The health professional must be attuned to this potential clash of needs and ensure that both parents and children are able to express their concerns and information requirements.

There is no doubt that healthcare consultations are a complex negotiation of different agendas, which are demanding even when they contain only two people. When a child has a long-standing illness and the parents are accustomed to communicating with health professionals without involving the child, embracing a different dynamic can be extremely challenging and the parents may not accept the position of 'bystander' very easily.[44] Alliances may already have been formed between the adults in the interaction, which can limit the amount the child then contributes.[35]

Parental attitudes and beliefs around health and illness are likely to have a significant impact upon how they parent their children, as well as the extent to which they encourage children to take responsibility when unwell or managing a condition. For example, is the prevailing belief within the family that only qualified professionals can manage their health and well-being? If so, this belief in the power of 'external' factors is likely to be adopted by other members of the family and, consequently, children may not see any role for themselves in the management of their condition. Similarly, during consultations parents often do not ask for the information they desire, or feel unable to disagree with health professionals.[2] Again, children may model this parental behaviour so that they too do not express their concerns or ask the questions that are important to them. Children are often socialised into a particular model of health behaviour which can be challenging to overcome, as with many other learnt behaviours.[10] It may be useful for the health professional to explore this with the family if they feel that this attitude could compromise the child's participation in treatment or the expression of their views on something that will affect them.

In order to include their children in discussions and decisions about health, parents will have to acknowledge that their child is an individual and may also have to accept that they cannot protect their children from everything. This can be exceptionally difficult for many parents and they may feel that their role as carer is under threat. They may also have previously worked hard to distance their child from their condition, where that condition is embarrassing or stigmatising, in order to spare their children anxiety or discomfort.[10] To reject this and encourage the child to participate in discussions and engage with decision-making may be very challenging for them and require substantial support from health professionals. Therefore, within a consultation there can be a conflict of agendas, which needs to be resolved before effective triadic communication can take place.

Summary of parent factors: some useful questions to consider

➤ What are the parents' views of health and illness?

➤ How much involvement do the parents themselves want in decision-making around their child's health?

➤ How much of the consultation is taken up with parental concerns?

➤ How are other decisions made in the family?

➤ Are there any reasons why the parents may be keen to distance the child from their condition?

➤ Is there a co-dependent relationship between the parent and child with respect to the child's illness?

Healthcare professional and environmental factors

There can be many reasons why health professionals fail to include children in their consultations and these factors will interact with one another. The environment within which modern medicine is often practised can be rushed and chaotic, with considerable time pressures on health professionals, parents and children. Hurried consultations on busy wards or in late-running clinics can be challenging for all parties, so that even if child participation is deemed desirable, reality is often different and paternalism prevails. When asked to describe how she included children in their asthma consultations, one nurse provided a response which may be familiar to many health professionals: 'I involve them by talking, questioning, handing out my own "simple guide to asthma", theoretically in choosing inhaler, checking inhaler technique, treatment plans. Time pressures mean that some of the theory goes out of the window'.[33] However, despite fears by many health professionals that the participation of a child will prolong the consultation, evidence suggests that this is not necessarily the case; two different studies have shown that when children spoke more in their consultations, the overall consultation time did not increase.[30,31]

There can be inconsistencies between the culture of different health professionals working within the same organisation, which can lead to differing approaches between departments, teams or even individuals. All individuals may well be working towards providing the best possible care for the child, but some may prioritise protecting the child while they do so, whereas others may subscribe more to the belief that the child has a right to be heard, even if that means sometimes the child may disagree with what is proposed. This may be an issue between disciplines, for example psychological team members may prioritise getting the child to take responsibility for managing their condition whereas surgical colleagues may be reluctant to inform the child fully about surgery in case it proves distressing and leads to refusal.

These attitudes are a major factor in determining the health professionals' approach to consultations, and health professionals themselves play a significant role in determining the extent of a child's involvement in a consultation. Previous literature has shown that where doctors have been supportive of a child's involvement, the child was more likely to speak, and was even more likely to speak where both adults were supportive.[32] However, some evidence suggests that the greater the number of adults present, the smaller the child's role in the consultation.[44]

The dominant communication model is one of consultation between the clinician and parent as 'proxy', with the child playing a marginal role. The reasons for this can be varied, but the health professional's communication skills are a key factor. Many health professionals feel more comfortable communicating with the parent than directly with the child. Uncertainties about the child's competence or worries that the child will refuse treatment can influence communication with them. Good communication skills are vital. Traditionally, textbooks on medical communication did not address communication with children and young people, although communication-skills training for health professionals is now much more inclusive, recognising the child-participation agenda.[49] Deering and Jennings suggest that asking why the child thinks they have come for the consultation can be illuminating, often revealing surprising misconceptions which are easily rectified.[50] Other simple strategies such as asking specific questions (e.g. 'Where does it hurt?') can be easier for children to answer than more general ones (e.g. 'How are you feeling?'). The use of some medical terminology may be appropriate – children do not want to be patronised or 'babied' – but may require an explanation so that they understand what is being discussed. Using such words without an explanation emphasises the health professional's status and minimises the child's involvement in the discussion. Going through symptoms in a checklist format can also minimise the child's active involvement, limiting them to one-word answers to confirm their presence or absence. Even then parents may answer for them.

Children are clear that their involvement must not be tokenistic. It is all too easy to ask a child's opinion only to continue with the proposed course of action whether or not the child is in favour. Some health professionals have even reported that, in effect, 'refusal isn't an option'.[42] While this may be unpalatable but necessary in life-threatening situations, in most other circumstances children's involvement can be facilitated so that it is meaningful, and that trust between child and the health professional is maintained. Health professionals who are open and communicative are highly regarded by children, while those who neglect their opinions are often criticised. Enabling a child's participation is certainly not an easy skill and it has been suggested that some health professionals feel poorly prepared to encounter empowered children. Participation may also require more 'effort' than simply issuing instructions. Even remembering to involve a long-standing child patient as they grow older may require effort; Garth *et al.* report a paediatrician saying, 'You do just talk to the parents when the children are babies and then as the children gradually grow up, you have to remember to bring the child into the conversation'.[35] The assumption that this inclusion will translate into increased consultation times has already been shown to be mistaken.

Summary of health professional factors: some useful questions to consider
➤ Does the surrounding environment encourage child participation? Consider privacy issues and time constraints. Can an alternative location be used?
➤ Am I worried that involving the child in discussions will increase consultation time?

➤ Is the child expressing a choice by withdrawing him/herself from discussions?
➤ Am I listening to what the child has to say?
➤ Am I involving the child in a tokenistic manner?
➤ Am I assuming the child is incompetent just because they disagree with what I am saying?
➤ Do I feel uncomfortable having my judgement questioned?

CONCLUSION

The participation of children and young people in consultations is subject to competing agendas from all who are involved in the discussions and can be affected by a multitude of factors. However, there are powerful arguments for including children in their healthcare, especially those who have chronic conditions, not least the demonstrable clinical and psychological benefits. As adults, we are expected to take responsibility for our health, but without training and preparation in childhood it is unlikely that this will happen effectively. Nova *et al.* have described children's interactions with health professionals as an 'apprenticeship, where the child learns to be a patient, both acquiring new medical information, and by interiorising a particular way of relating to the doctor'.[51] It is clear that health consultations offer a golden opportunity to engage with children, and health professionals play a crucial role in working with children and parents to lay the foundations for future participation in their healthcare.

ACKNOWLEDGEMENTS

Thank you to Sarah Redsell for our useful discussions around this topic. Thank you also to Debra Forster for her helpful clinical input.

REFERENCES

1 Coyne I. Consultation with children in hospital: children, parents' and nurses' perspectives. *J Clin Nurs.* 2006; **15**: 61–71.
2 Jackson C, Cheater FM, Reid I. A systematic review of decision support needs of parents making child health decisions. *Health Expect.* 2008; **11**: 232–51.
3 Alderson P, Montgomery J. What about me? *Health Serv J.* 1996; 22–4.
4 Eiser C. It's OK having asthma . . . young children's beliefs about illness. *Prof Nurse.* 1991; **6**(6); 342–45.
5 Department of Health. *5 A Day.* London: Department of Health; 2003. Available at: www. dh.gov.uk/en/Publichealth/Healthimprovement/FiveADay/index.htm (accessed 10 June 2010).
6 Department of Health. *Alcohol Misuse: what we are doing.* London: Department of Health; 2009. Available at: http://webarchive.nationalarchives.gov.uk/+/www.dh.gov. uk/en/Publichealth/Healthimprovement/Alcoholmisuse/DH_085349 (accessed 10 June 2010).

7 National Institute for Health and Clinical Excellence (NICE). *Four Commonly Used Methods to Increase Physical Activity: brief interventions in primary care, exercise referral schemes, pedometers and community-based exercise programmes for walking and cycling*. London: NICE; 2003. Available at: www.nice.org.uk/guidance/PHI2 (accessed 10 June 2010).

8 Bandura A. Perceived self-efficacy in the exercise of personal agency. *Psychol Bull Br Psychol Soc*. 1989; Oct: 411–24.

9 Worthy A. Promoting emotional and social development. *Spotlight*. 2005; **6**: 1–4.

10 Bury M, Gabe J, Olumide G, *et al. Patients as Partners: children and the National Health Service*. University of London: Royal Holloway; 2004; pp. 1–63.

11 Bee H, Boyd D. *The Developing Child*. 10th ed. New York: Allyn & Bacon; 2003.

12 Pantell R, Lewis C. Talking with children: how to improve the process and outcomes of medical care. *Med Encounter*. 1993; **10**: 3–7.

13 Roter D, Frankel R. Quantitative and qualitative approaches to the evaluation of the medical dialogue. *Soc Sci Med*. 1992; **34**(10): 1097–103.

14 Wissow LS, Roter D, Bauman LJ, *et al*. Patient–provider communication during the emergency department care of children with asthma. *Med Care*. 1998; **36**(10): 1439–50.

15 Department of Health (DH). *The National Service Framework for Children, Young People and Maternity Services*. London: DH; 2004.

16 Boylan P. *Children's Voices Project*. London: Commission for Health Improvement, Department of Health; 2004; 1–37.

17 Buford T. School-age children with asthma and their parents: relationships with health care providers. *Issues Compr Pediatr Nurs*. 2005; **28**(3): 153–62.

18 Theunissen N, Vogels T, Koopman H, *et al*. The proxy problem: child report versus parent report in health-related quality of life. *Qual Life Res*. 1998; **7**: 387–97.

19 McGrath P, McAlpine L. Psychological perspectives on pediatric pain. *J Pediatr*. 2003; **122**(5:2): S2–S8.

20 Rushforth H. Practitioner review: communicating with hospitalised children: review and application of research pertaining to children's understanding of illness. *J Child Psychol Psyc*. 1999; **40**(5): 683–91.

21 Tieffenberg J, Wood E, Alonso A, *et al*. A randomised field trial of ACINDES: a child-centred training model for children with chronic illness (asthma and epilepsy). *J Urban Health*. 2000; **77**(2): 280–97.

22 McPherson AC, Glazebrook C, Forster D, *et al*. A randomized, controlled trial of an interactive educational computer package for children with asthma. *Pediatrics*. 2006; **117**(4): 1046–54.

23 Lewis M, Lewis G. Consequences of empowering children to care for themselves. *Pediatrician*. 1990; **17**: 63–7.

24 McQuaid E, Kopel S, Klein R, *et al*. Medication adherence in pediatric asthma: reasoning, responsibility and behavior. *J Pediatr Psychol*. 2003; **28**(5): 323–33.

25 Guevara J, Wolf F, Grum G, *et al*. Effects of educational interventions for self-management of asthma in children and adolescents: systematic review and meta-analysis. *Brit Med J*. 2003; **326**: 1308–9.

26 Schmidt S, Peterson C, Bullinger M. Coping with chronic disease from the perspective of

children and adolescents – a conceptual framework and its implications for participation. *Child Care Health and Dev.* 2003; (1): 63–75.

27 Lewis G, Lewis M. Children's health-related decision making. *Health Educ Q.* 1982; 9(2–3): 225–37.

28 Lewis G, Rachelefsky G, Lewis M, *et al.* A randomised trial of A.C.T. (Asthma Care Training) for kids. *Pediatrics.* 1984; **74**(4): 478–86.

29 Tates K, Meeuwesen L. Doctor–parent–child communication: a (re)view of the literature. *Soc Sci Med.* 2001; **52**: 839–51.

30 Wassmer E, Minnaar G, Adbdel AN, *et al.* How do paediatricians communicate with children and parents? *Acta Pædiatr.* 2004; **93**: 1501–6.

31 van Dulmen A. Children's contributions to pediatric outpatient encounters. *Pediatrics.* 1998; **102**(3): 563–8.

32 Tates K, Elbers E, Meeuwesen L, *et al.* Doctor–parent–child relationships: a 'pas de trois'. *Patient Educ Couns.* 2002; **48**: 5–14.

33 McPherson AC, Redsell SA. Factors affecting children's involvement in asthma consultations: a questionnaire survey of general practitioners and primary care asthma nurses. *Prim Care Respir J.* 2009; **18**(1): 15–20.

34 Alderson P, Sutcliffe K, Curtis K. Children as partners with adults in their medical care. *Arch Dis Child.* 2006; **91**: 300–3.

35 Garth B, Murphy G, Reddihough D. Perceptions of participation: child patients with a disability in the doctor–parent–child partnership. *Patient Educ Couns.* 2009; **74**: 45–52.

36 Cahill P, Papageorgiou A. Video analysis of communication in paediatric consultations in primary care. *Brit J Gen Pract.* Nov 2007; 866–71.

37 Bibace R, Walsh M. Development of children's concepts of illness. *Pediatrics.* 1980; **66**(6): 912–17.

38 Charman T, Chandiramani S. Children's understanding of physical illness and psychological states. *Psychol Health.* 1995; **10**: 145–53.

39 Wood D. *How Children Think and Learn.* Oxford: Blackwell; 1998.

40 Meadows S. Cognitive development. In: Bryant P, Colman A (editors). *Developmental Psychology.* Harrow: Longman; 1995.

41 Smith P, Gowie H, Blades M. *Understanding Children's Development.* Oxford: Blackwell; 2003.

42 Coyne I. Children's participation in consultations and decision-making at health service level: a review of the literature. *Int J Nurs Stud.* 2008; **45**: 1682–9.

43 Angst D, Deatrick J. Involvement in health care decisions: parents and children with chronic illness. *J Fam Nurs.* 1996; **2**(2): 174–94.

44 Pyörälä E. The participation roles of children and adolescents in the dietary counseling of diabetics. *Patient Educ Couns.* 2004; **55**(3): 385–95.

45 Runeson I, Enskär K, Elander G, *et al.* Professionals' perceptions of children's participation in decision-making in healthcare. *J Clin Nurs.* 2001; **10**: 70–8.

46 Tates K, Meeuwesen L, Elbers E, *et al.* 'I've come for his throat': roles and identities in doctor–parent–child communication. *Child Care Health and Dev.* 2002; **28**(1): 109–16.

47 Ohanion N. Information needs of child and adolescent cancer patients and their parents. *J Pediatr Onco Nurs.* 1993; **7**(2): 135–46.

48 Hendricson W, Wood P, Hidalgo H, *et al.* Implementation of individualised patient education for Hispanic children with asthma. *Patient Educ Couns.* 1996; **29**: 155–65.

49 Beresford B, Sloper P. Chronically ill adolescents' experiences of communicating with doctors: a qualitative study. *J Adolesc Health.* 2003; **33**(3): 172–9.

50 Deering C, Jennings D. Communicating with children and adolescents. *Am J Nurs.* 2002; **102**(3): 34–41.

51 Nova C, Vegni E, Moja A. The physician–patient–parent communication: a qualitative perspective on the child's contribution. *Patient Educ Couns.* 2005; **58**: 327–33.

CHAPTER 3

The third voice in the consultation

Patricia Cahill

INTRODUCTION

A child's healthcare encounter usually entails the meeting of at least three people: a child, a parent and a health professional. The talk in these triads, when successful, has been likened to 'a pas de trois', a delicate interplay between the participants.[1] However, in most of these meetings there may well be more than three sets of dynamics in orchestration, from outside the room as well as from within: those of absent family, school teachers, peers and even the state.[2] Health professionals conducting their part in the interaction have to bear in mind rules of confidentiality, assessment of competency, guidance on the safeguarding of the young patient, while building rapport and trust, to arrive at a functional harmony.

Multiparty discussions are inherently more complex that those between just two people, particularly if every individual's feelings and opinions are to be taken into account. This does not always happen when the individual is a child. A child has relatively little say in medical dialogue.[3,4] Two studies from the UK, where the health professionals were doctors, found the child's portion of the total communication in the consultation was 4% and 5.4% respectively.[5,6] Governmental and professional guidelines are urging more child-centred care.[7,8] Children's lack of involvement in their health consultations can leave them feeling marginalised.[9] There is evidence that a child's active involvement in his or her own healthcare is beneficial to some of the outcomes.[10] Some children have requested more of a voice.[11] However, whether the desire to have a say in medical consultations holds for all children is unclear. There are those who may prefer an adult to speak on their behalf. One of the skills that a health professional needs is identifying which children want to talk.

EVIDENCE ON COMMUNICATION IN CONSULTATIONS WITH CHILDREN

Evidence elucidating these triadic encounters is available from the Netherlands undertaken by Tates and her colleagues.[1,3,12–14] They examined recordings of paediatric consultations taken from an archive. These recordings made between the 1970s and 1990s featured a child (average age of eight years), a carer and a doctor. The sample included audio and audio visual data. They were subjected to a series of analyses. This revealed that the child's quantifiable participation in the consultations has increased over the years, with the doctors becoming progressively more child-centred.[12] The children were observed to be capable of contributing substantially to the work of the consultations and not just be involved in a jokey or social way.[13] The doctors would particularly try to involve older children.[1,12] The researchers noted that the children's parents tended not to make a similar accommodation for age. This finding led the authors to suggest that in order to promote a child's involvement in consultations a health professional should make the desirability of this explicit.[12] The analyses showed how children predominately end up voiceless at the end of consultations, even if at the beginning the clinician had tried to include them.[1,14] The child might be involved in history taking and examination but be excluded from treatment and planning. This situation is exacerbated when either the doctor or the parent is supportive of child involvement and most marked when neither is supportive.[1] The Dutch researchers were able to demonstrate how the situation of the adult speaking for the child is institutional, a social co-construction with all parties implicated in creating and maintaining the situation.[14] Furthermore, the analyses confirmed how important is the adult carers' support and permission for child involvement in the medical encounter.[1,12]

The children's parents have considerable power in these interactions.[15] The health professional has a degree of control being in a position to invite participants to speak or ask a parent to allow a child to speak.[12,15] However, if such a request is resisted by a carer this is problematic for the health professional; talking with a child when it appears to be against a carer's wishes may be considered impolite.[16] Going against the grain of a parent's wishes can cause awkwardness and further detriment to the child's participation, if it leads to tension in the communication.

PRIMARY CARE AND PAEDIATRIC CONSULTATIONS

Most children in the UK are seen in primary care at some time in their childhood and a large majority of contacts between children and health professionals occur in this setting.[17] Most primary care professionals have considerable experience in dealing with child patients, particularly with the types of problems that present or are managed in the community. Secondary care looks after children who need their specialist dedicated service, frequently in conjunction with primary care colleagues. Paediatric case vignettes taken from the primary care setting in the UK will be used here to demonstrate some observations on multiparty dynamics. These stories are not reproductions of any actual cases but rather an amalgamation of many similar ones encountered in routine practice.

Greetings

> **CASE 1:** Aaron
>
> Dr Brown visited a three-year-old child at home. She had been told that the child, Aaron, was too unwell to be moved. She was met by four adults who accompanied her into the sitting room where a child, pink and comfortable, was lying on the couch. There were two more women already sitting beside the child. After introducing herself Dr Brown gestured towards Aaron, while looking at one of the standing adults saying softly, 'Aaron?' A man replied, 'Yes'. None of the adults introduced themselves. The doctor added, 'Are you all Aaron's relatives?' The man who had already spoken said, 'I'm Dad, this is Mum and Grandma', as he pointed in the direction of the seated women. The three other adults left the room at this point and shut the door.

Dr Brown is confronted by a host of people. She introduces herself so that they know who she is. She then goes on to try and establish who the other people are. The doctor could be viewed by the family as an entity, rather than as a guest, therefore not requiring the usual exchange of social greetings. It is very likely that Aaron's illness is causing anxiety.[18,19] Dr Brown's first priority is Aaron's well-being. Too many people in the room may impede her ability to assess and relate to him. Aaron and his parents may also need some privacy and a confiding environment. Dr Brown addresses this issue by asking if the assembled people are relatives, thus indirectly indicating that it may be inappropriate for non-relatives to be present. Three of the adults leave. The grandmother stays. This indicates that the grandmother thinks it appropriate to do so. The doctor cannot really tell for sure if Aaron and his parents share the same viewpoint but they do not say otherwise. The status of grandparents differs greatly between different family settings. The doctor here allows a silent negotiation to occur within the family, and she accepts the grandmother's attendance following the family's lead.

Greeting patients in the clinic is slightly different. The patient and the family might not feel as comfortable as they would in their own home. This is the health professional's 'territory'. It falls to the health professional to relax the patient and any accompanying carers. In this situation, the health professional still needs to know who is who and what their relationship is to the child, in particular identifying who has parental responsibility. Usually, only relevant 'others' would accompany a child to a medical appointment, so the problem of a crowded consulting room is less likely to occur. In primary care, as in most clinic-based settings, the patients arrive and wait in a waiting room. Children should be seen promptly, if possible, as waiting can be tedious for them and may cause them to worry.[20] The child and his carer are either summoned to the clinic room by a buzzer or met and greeted in the waiting room.

The greeting is usually most successful if it is friendly and warm.[21] Children may not initially want to say anything, until they are familiar with the health professional.

Seating

The seating arrangement and positioning of individuals in multiparty consultations has an impact on the ensuing discussion.[6,22] A detailed analysis of a series of consultations conducted by general practitioners concluded that the most favourable seating arrangement for consulting with a parent and a child, aged six to twelve years, was for them to sit in a triangular arrangement, the parties being an equal distant apart.[6] This means there is no adult acting as a barrier preventing child access to the clinician. Each person can see the other two by a slight turn of the head. Three-way talk can easily occur. True multiparty talk is facilitated, rather than conversation between two of the participants, which a linear arrangement of chairs might promote. If two people come with the child, such as a mother and father, the triangle of seats can be widened to a square.

Younger children might want to sit on the parent's knee.[22] Some children may want to put a little distance between themselves and the health professional, so flexibility and sensitivity to individual children's needs is required.

CASE 2: Peter

A nurse practitioner (NP) collects a child patient from the waiting room and stands in the open door of the consulting room.

NP: Do come in, Peter, Mrs Black. [Mrs Black and Peter walk through the door.]

NP: Peter, would you like to sit there? [Looking at Peter and pointing towards Peter's chair.]

The NP, using gesture, gaze and voice, requests that Peter sits in the chair next to her.

Initiating the consultation

CASE 3: Michael

Michael, aged six years, and his mother are seeing the NP.

NP: Now, Michael, what can I do for you? [Looks towards Michael and away from his mother.]

Michael: [While looking at the NP he does not answer for 4 seconds] Uuuum. I don't know [Michael turns to his mother]. Mum?

Mum: I'm really worried. He was very unwell last night and I really think something is going on. I took his temperature and it was sky-high.

NP: Okay, we'll check that in a minute. I will just ask Michael to tell me how he is feeling if that is okay, to try and understand more. [Looks at mother, then looks

> down at Michael, stooping down to get at eye level with him.] Now, Michael,
> how are you feeling at the moment?
>
> Michael: [8 seconds' pause] All right.
>
> NP: Do you feel bad any where?
>
> Michael: [4 seconds' pause] No.
>
> After further talk of symptoms and gathering of information, the consultation continues.
>
> NP: And what did you have for breakfast this morning?
>
> Michael: [2 seconds' pause] I had two Weetabix and toast.
>
> Mum: [Speaking over Michael] He's a good eater even when he is ill.
>
> NP: [Looks at mother and smiles in response, then looks at Michael] May I take
> your temperature and look in your ears and in your mouth?
>
> Michael: [Pause] Yes.
>
> NP: Okay with you, Mum? [Looking up at mother.]

Addressing Michael

After all have greeted and seated, the NP asks Michael what she can do for him. She asks his mother for permission to speak with Michael and explains why this is important.[12] The NP gets down to eye level. This action is commonly recommended in communication with children. Michael does not answer the initial question posed to him but passes the responsibility on to his mother. It is common for a health professional to ask the child what the presenting problem is but it is not usual for the parent to answer.[23] The NP here shows that it is Michael she is addressing rather than his mother; she does this by using his name, looking at him and making sure that the mother can see that she is doing so. If children are actively invited to speak there is a greater chance that they will. The compliant child is the least powerful member in the consultation.[15] So, it is important for the health professional to have actively made this selection of the child. Having been addressed like this Michael is more likely to speak later in the consultation.[14,23]

Giving Michael time to respond

When a child does reply he may leave a much longer pause before answering a question than an adult would. It can seem as if this pause is uncomfortably long. Some parents or carers have a tendency to speak in an attempt to 'help out'. The clinician may also, because of the length of this pause, think a child is not going to say anything and prematurely look to the carer, thus inviting her to answer instead. The NP here makes it easier for Michael to gather his thoughts for his response by maintaining her gaze in his direction, holding the floor for him and giving him plenty of time. If his mother did answer for him immediately and then a second question was directed at Michael, his mother would be likely to remain silent and wait for Michael to answer. Without having verbal clues, the NP has to use sensitivity and judgement, reading Michael's face and body language to ensure she is assisting him in participating in the consultation but not pressurising him.

Mum has her say

In this consultation, the mother has an opportunity to express her concerns early on in the discourse when she tells the NP that she is really worried about Michael. It has been shown that if parents are not able to express concerns early on in the consultation and the clinician has been successful in engaging in clinician–child talk, the adult is likely to interrupt.[6] Once the adult has interrupted in this way the consultation is likely to revert to adult–adult talk, with the child excluded from then on.[1,6]

Mum keeping the consultation on the 'right' track

Open questions are usually the best way to get an unbiased opinion but children's answers can be influenced by previous discussions with parents. Children sometimes attempt to give the 'correct answer' when asked a question, falling in line with the parental view.[6] Some children can find very open questions more challenging in the clinic environment than slightly more closed ones, such as here. Michael seems to find it easier to answer the NP about what he had for breakfast. After an initial reply, a short string of phases regarding this meal ensues. Mum breaks in to keep the consultation on track. Michael is saying that he eats well. She is more experienced with medical situations than Michael, aware that eating well is a sign of good health and she may be concerned that this could mean that the NP will then not take her concerns so seriously. Mum may want some control of the consultation.[15] Parents admit to worrying about what their child might say that could diminish the validity of the decision to consult and parents sometimes upgrade the children's symptoms to 'clarify' the problem to the health professional.[6]

The next stage of this consultation is the examination. This can be a special phase in a consultation where the health professional has more direct contact with the child.[12]

Michael expressing his concerns

Children are very rarely heard to express their concerns in consultation. They can be encouraged to do so, especially towards the end when the pressure of the business is finished.

NP: Michael, is there anything you are worried about? [Soft voice, unhurried pace.]
          [Long pause of 20 seconds.]
NP: Is there anything you want to ask?
Mum: You can ask her, Michael.
Michael: [Pause] Will I have to have a blood test? My sister says it will really hurt.
NP: No, Michael, we don't need to do a blood test. [Pause] They are only done if absolutely necessary.

Children can have worries that might be very difficult for them to voice. Here the NP gives plenty of encouragement and time. Mum adds her support.[1]

In this case, the health professional uses clear, simple language throughout the consultation and breaks the information into small chunks. Michael is taken seriously and not patronised. He is able to talk to the NP about the possibility of a blood test.

Children may not mention concerns they have, or may not wish to share them with an unfamiliar adult. It can be helpful to remember that children often think in terms of their world.[6] A child might well be worrying about something that a clinician would not expect, guess at or ever imagine.

MOTHERS, FATHERS, GRANDPARENTS

The majority of children are brought to see health professionals with one person and this is often the mother. Fathers and grandparents, as well as other carers, might accompany the child and who this is may reflect the domestic situation. If the primary carer has not been able to come, his or her ideas will require consideration. The present carer may overtly say that Dad, Mum or some other significant person has been unable to attend. The health professional may glean this information from the nature of the conversation, body language and this person's interaction with the child. It may be that he or she does not appear to have the knowledge that would be expected from a carer. If this is the case, the professional seeing the child needs to be very sure about the role of this person and their relationship to the child. Are they in a position to give consent on the child's behalf where necessary in the absence of the parent? Should they be there, privy to the interview? If there is any suspicion that they should not be there, then there is a problem regarding parental responsibility and confidentiality. For example, a disapproving grandparent bringing a grandchild without parental knowledge to get 'a proper check up'.

Another scenario might be one parent bringing the child on instruction from the other. The health professional has to negotiate with someone not in the room. When the carer does not really know what is going on with the child, this can be a chance for the child to speak. However, even in this circumstance, when the information is collected from the child, he still may be excluded from the rest of the consultation.[24]

Both parents attending

Sometimes two main carers will come with a child, for example both parents. This could be because it is family custom to do so, or possibly because of language difficulties. Often the primary carer takes the lead. Both parents being present could mean that the consultation is viewed as 'more serious'. It may be due to the perceived need for extra support or a major concern. It could also be as a result of a prior problem, such as 'a wished for' referral not being arranged; the second parent may be there as a reinforcement. The dynamics are more complex for the health professional to navigate, the more parties that are present. The health professional is unlikely to be aware of any issues between the couple that might be cordial or destructive. With more adults present the child may be slightly intimidated and less likely to speak.

There are more speakers available to talk on the child's behalf. The health professional might also be intimidated. It is important to try to discover all the agendas and to be ruled by the guiding principle of conducting the consultation in the best interest of the child. If there is a point of contention with the medical care this can be seen as an opportunity for discussion.

Siblings

A sibling might be attending a consultation with a brother or sister as a second patient or because there was nowhere else to leave him. An audience like this can be embarrassing for the child patient. Potentially confidential information could be divulged and used against him later! The child patient may be reticent in front of his brother or sister. This increases the challenge for the clinician of building rapport. Bored siblings can be noisy and distracting for everyone and result in the whole consultation being rushed with increased levels of tension. On a more optimistic note a child might find her sibling supportive, a confidence boost with a positive impact on the consultation. It could induce more sibling care and understanding for the 'unwell' family member.

Can my friend come too?

Health centres can be intimidating places for young people. The Royal College of General Practitioners and the Royal College of Nursing have for many years now been working on an initiative to make this a less common occurrence and for young people to feel welcome.[25,26] A young person might elect to bring a friend when attending a medical appointment. This potentially means that the patient is being supported by a close, like-minded person, but could also mean peer pressure and compromised confidentiality. The health professional will want to be sure it is the patient's ideas they are discussing and that she is not being coerced in any way. These friends may have had extensive discussions before this visit and be very much of one agenda. How the consultation is handled may have wider implications if reported back to their friends, sending positive health messages or otherwise to their community. Some health professionals may feel concerned regarding being alone with one or two young people in case there are any misunderstandings that have later repercussions. Ways to deal with this problem need consideration. Young people appreciate being treated with respect and sensitivity, building up a relationship and rapport with health services. A young person making appointments on her own or with a friend may mean that she is in considerable difficulty.[27] Making the appointment should be as easy as possible and sensible judgements should be used on behalf of the booking staff not to impede access to health advice.

Seeing children alone

It is a very unusual situation for a primary school child to attend a medical consultation completely alone, although it can happen, for example, in a boarding school. The General Medical Council's guidance for doctors communicating with children states that doctors should make it clear that they are available to see children and young people on their own, without giving the impression that they need to be with a parent to access the service. They do not suggest any age limit for this and further add that the doctors should think carefully about the effect the presence of a chaperone can have on a young person's ability to be frank in asking for help.[7]

CASE 4: Mary

Mary is 14 years old. She has been brought to the doctor by her mother because she has been experiencing lower abdominal pain. Mum is worried this might be appendicitis. She feels she knows her daughter well and they have a good relationship. She knows that Mary started her periods over a year ago and that they are regular. She is proud of Mary for doing well at school. She is very protective of Mary and thinks she is 'young' for her age. Mary looks well and examination of her abdomen is normal.

Mary has a boyfriend and they are sexually active. She is terrified that her mother might find out. If she were to be asked about her periods in front of her mother she would say they were regular rather than that she had missed the last two. Mary may only admit to being worried that she is pregnant if she has the chance to see the doctor alone.

Involve the child in the whole consultation

A young person with lower abdominal pain like this could have early appendicitis. Appendicitis is a condition that can be difficult to diagnose accurately in the early stages. Based on the history and examination available, the decision might be made for Mary to go home. Usual practice in this case would be to ask the patient to monitor the symptoms and to come back if things got worse.[28] A young person of Mary's age can usually be actively involved throughout the entire consultation, including the decisions about follow-up.[29] Thus, Mary is taking some responsibility for her condition rather than it all resting with her mother.

However, in Mary's situation there is the possibility that she is pregnant. If she were, her pain could be a serious complication of this. A prominently displayed poster in the waiting room, or leaflets directed at young people, may guide her to better know that she is able to be seen without her mother.[25,30]

Routinely ask parents to 'step out for a moment'

For Mary's optimal care the doctor needs to know of possible pregnancy in this consultation. If she believes that to make a proper safe assessment she needs to see Mary alone, she will need to request this. If it was her practice to ask the parents routinely to step out for a few moments when consulting with 14-year-old girls, then the opportunity to speak with Mary alone and hopefully gain her trust and confidence could easily and seamlessly be achieved. If mother has never been asked to leave the room before, she may be surprised and possibly resistant; however, she is unlikely to refuse, especially if the request is made in a politely assertive manor. She is almost certainly going to wonder what is discussed and how to handle her inquiry is an issue Mary will have to deal with.

When alone with Mary the doctor can assess her competence as the discussion continues. She can offer Mary confidentially and privacy but with the proviso that she might have to share information with others if it were in Mary's best interest. Younger people, like most adults, understand this and respond well to such open, honest, respectful dialogue.

The doctor explores whether it would be appropriate for Mary to discuss her worries with her mother. She may be able to help her to do so. Whether Mary is pregnant or not, this is an opportunity to build trust. The guiding principle is Mary's welfare.

Young people as parents

CASE 5: Liam and Sonia

Liam is 15 years old and living with his mother. He has recently become a father to Jake. He has had a troubled time at school with periods of exclusion as a younger child. He is now in school, trying to do well. He is chuffed about being a father and wants the best for Jake. Liam is very worried about Jake having immunisations. He is particularly concerned about the whooping cough element. He believes that it would give Jake epilepsy, which Liam has himself. Sonia is also 15 years old and is Jake's mother. She lives with her own mother, Marie, and baby Jake. She is doing well after the birth.

Liam, Sonia and Marie bring Jake to see the practice nurse, Sally, for his first immunisation. Marie is holding Jake. Sally hears Liam's concerns. She checks the contraindications list to the vaccine in front of the family. She takes Liam seriously and then is able to go on and discuss with the family the pros and cons of having the vaccine. Sonia does not say very much but the nurse actively asks her if she is happy about Jake having the immunisations. The parents and Marie agree for the vaccination to go ahead. The nurse asks who would like to hold Jake for the immunisation looking at Sonia, who says she will do so. After the immunisation Sonia books to see the nurse again for contraceptive advice. Liam and Sonia found Sally, the nurse, approachable and friendly and they felt relaxed. They felt empowered to share their opinions and to negotiate Jake's care.

The subject of adolescent parenthood is complex. Liam and Sonia have to manage looking after their child while still making the transition from adolescence to adulthood themselves. The well-being of Jake is everyone's priority. Health professionals have been criticised by adolescent parents for being judgemental and 'looking down their noses'.[31] Jake needs to be able to access health provision in the same way as a baby with older parents could, and for this to occur it is helpful if Jake's parents feel that the health professionals are approachable. The dynamics of the interaction between the nurse and the young parents start well before they bring Jake in to her room. Some young people find receptionists in healthcare settings overbearing. This could be as a result of mismatching stereotypes on both their parts.[31]

These young parents have been listened to. Both Liam and Sonia have to be involved in decisions about Jake. Sally, the nurse, treats the couple with the same respect she would give any parent in a way that is appropriate for them. She may temper what she says to allow for the fact they are young and do not have the same experience with words or attending health settings as parents twice their age. She shows a realisation that these parents may need her to be accommodating, flexible, and to give them time. Sally also ensures Marie is onboard as she is a major support for Jake's parents. Marie may have other children, have ideas of her own on child rearing and 'look after' Jake too much. She may not be ready to be a grandmother or she may indeed want to have more children herself. The nurse's behaviour in the consultation builds the parents' confidence. A relationship of trust and respect has been created which can be developed in further meetings. Contraception is a priority and Sonia feels able to return to discuss this with Sally. The building of rapport makes it easier for Sally and other members of the primary care team to be a source of ongoing support.

Social services, as well as other dedicated professionals such as midwives, health visitors and educators, may have considerable input into this family. The nurse may need to communicate with the wider team. Liam's involvement and interest in Jake's young life is beneficial for Jake. Although Liam and Sonia's romantic relationship may be perishable, Liam having an ongoing connection will be advantageous for all three. Young fathers can feel isolated from their children. Liam has a strong desire to provide the best life for Jake. Sensitive handling in situations such as this can have long-term implications and rewards.

CONCLUSION

Every health encounter is unique because the people involved in it are individuals. We have taken a broad-brush approach here to some complex issues. The principle guiding the health professional, however complicated the consultation, is to act in the best interest of the child. Important skills include active listening, as well as being sensitive to children as patients and those close to them. All the parties in these paediatric consultations, including the children themselves, may not anticipate the child acting in true partnership with the adults in line with age and ability. The health professional is in a position to tune the other participants in to an awareness of this and conduct the consultation in such a way that it takes on a child-centred focus, allowing the child to be a true player in their healthcare.

REFERENCES

1 Tates K, Elbers E, Meeuwesen L, *et al.* Doctor–parent–child relationships: 'a pas de trois'. *Patient Educ Couns.* 2002; **48**(1): 5–14.

2 Innes A, Campion P, Griffiths F. Complex consultations and the 'edge of chaos'. *Brit J Gen Pract.* 2005; **55**: 47–52.

3 Tates K, Meeuwesen L. Doctor–parent–child communication: a review of the literature. *Soc Sci Med.* 2001; **52**(6): 839–51.

4 Cahill P, Papageorgiou A. Triadic communication in the primary care paediatric consultation: a review of the literature. *Brit J Gen Pract.* 2007; **57**: 904–11.

5 Wassmer E, Minnaar G, Abdel Aal N, *et al.* How do paediatricians communicate with children and parents? *Acta Pæditr.* 2004; **93**: 1501–6.

6 Cahill P, Papageorgiou A. Video analysis of communication in paediatric consultations in primary care. *Brit J Gen Pract.* 2007; **57**: 866.

7 General Medical Council (GMC). *0–18 Years: guidance for all doctors.* London: GMC; 2007.

8 Department of Health. *Transforming Community Services: ambition, action, and achievement. Transforming services for children, young people and their families.* London: DoH; 2009.

9 Young B, Dixon-Woods M, Windridge K, *et al.* Managing communication with young people who have a potentially life threatening chronic illness: qualitative study of patients and parents. *Brit Med J.* 2003; **326**: 305–10.

10 Lewis C, Rachelefsky G, Lewis M, *et al.* A randomized trial of A.C.T. (Asthma Care Training) for kids. *Pediatrics.* 1984; **74**(4): 478–86.

11 Boylan P. *Children's Voices Project: feedback from children and young people about their experience and expectations of health care.* Commission for Health Improvement, National Health Service England and Wales; 2004. Available at: www.cqc.org.uk/_db/_documents/04012717.pdf (accessed 10 June 2010).

12 Tates K, Meeuwesen L. Let Mum have her say: turntaking in doctor–parent–child communication. *Patient Educ Couns.* 2000; **40**(2): 151–62.

13 Tates K, Meeuwesen L, Bensing J, *et al.* (2002a). Joking or decision-making? Affective and Instrumental behaviour in doctor–parent–child communication. *Psychol Health.* 2002; **17**(3): 281–95.

14 Tates K, Meeuwesen L, Bensing J. 'I've come about his throat': roles and identities in doctor–parent–child communication. *Child Care Health and Dev.* 2002; **28**(1): 109–16.

15 Aronsson K, Rundström B. Child discourse and parental control in pediatric consultations. *Text.* 1988; **8**: 159–89.

16 Aronsson K, Rundstrom B. Cats, dogs and sweets in the clinical negotiation of reality: on politeness and coherence in pediatric discourse. *Lang Soc.* 1989; **18**: 483–504.

17 Peter L. Services for children: primary care. *Brit Med J.* 1993; **307**: 117–20.

18 Wyke S, Hewison J, Russell I. Respiratory illness in children: what makes parents decide to consult? *Brit J Gen Pract.* 1990; **40**: 226–9.

19 Martin E, Russell D, Goodwin S, *et al.* Why patients consult and what happens when they do. *Brit Med J.* 1991; **303**: 289–92.

20 Curtis K, Liabo K, Roberts H, *et al.* Consulted but not heard: a qualitative study of young people's views of their local health service. *Health Expect.* 2004; **7**: 149–56.

21 Cook P. 'Will it hurt?' Children and medical settings. In: Milner P, Carolin B. *Time to Listen to Children: personal and professional communication.* London: Routledge; 1999.

22 Hart C, Bain J. *Child Care in General Practice.* London: Churchill Livingstone; 1989.

23 Stivers T. Negotiating who presents the problem: next speaker selection in pediatric encounters. *J Comm.* 2001; **51**(2): 252–82.

24 Pantell R, Stewart T, Dias J, *et al.* Physician communication with children and parents. *Pediatrics.* 1982; **70**(3): 396–402.

25 Department of Health, Royal College of Nursing, The National Youth Agency, Brook. *'You're Welcome' Quality Criteria: making health services more young people friendly*. London: DH Publications; 2007.

26 Jacobson L. The RCGP Adolescent Task Group reaches its teenage years. *Brit J Gen Pract*. 2007; **57**(542): 749.

27 Wrate R. Talking to adolescents. In: Myerscough P, Ford M (editors). *Talking With Patients: keys to good communication*. Oxford: Oxford Medical Publications; 1996.

28 Neighbour R. *The Inner Consultation*. Lancaster: Kluwer Academic Publishers; 1987.

29 Eminson M, Coupe W. GPs communication with children and adolescents. *Context*. 2000; **50**: 3.

30 Royal College of Nursing, Royal College of General Practitioners. *Getting it Right for Teenagers in your Practice*. London: Royal College of General Practitioners and the Royal College of Nursing; 2002.

31 Department for Children, Schools and Families (DCSF). *Getting Maternity Services Right for Teenagers and Young Fathers*. Nottingham: DCSF Publications; 2008.

CHAPTER 4

Involving children: how to do it

Anne Willmott

INTRODUCTION

Previous chapters have looked at children's development and understanding at different ages and why their involvement is important (Chapters 2 and 3). This chapter will discuss practical techniques for promoting the involvement of children in the consultation process, and how to make our communication with children and families more effective. Research has shown that in doctor–parent–child consultations only 6–14% of interactions occur between doctor and child, most of which is limited to social chit-chat.[1] This means that for about 90% of the consultation both adults ignore the child. Clearly, we have a long way to go in our efforts to involve children.

This raises the question of why we should bother. If most consultations with children ignore the child but appear to have a satisfactory outcome, why should we even try? Do most professionals speak almost exclusively to the mother (here used as shorthand for whichever carer or parent comes with the child) because it is unnecessary, inefficient or impossible to speak directly to the child?

As described in Chapter 1, the attitudes of health professionals and the institutions they work in have evolved towards greater participation. This change has been encouraged by formal guidance, recommendations and by changes in the laws affecting children.[2-4] In order to do this, even young children need to be actively involved in the consultation process. As the health professional, we set the tone for the consultation – if we take a lead in involving the child, the carer is more likely to include them as well.

In addition to a rights-based motivation for involving children, I think there are a number of other reasons:

➤ it is the child who is our patient – it is good to remind ourselves, the parents and the child of this
➤ an involved child is less disruptive

➤ an involved child is more likely to cooperate with any intervention
➤ children involved in planning and decisions can have better outcomes[5]
➤ I am a paediatrician – I think it is more fun!

The techniques and principles described apply to anyone dealing with children and families, and will be relevant to any health professional, whatever their role.

THE CONSULTATION PROCESS

A model of the consultation for all practitioners

- Interpret prior knowledge about the patient.
- Set your goals for the consultation.
- Gather sufficient information to make a provisional diagnosis, using a biopsychosocial model of disease.
- Discover the patient's ideas, concerns and expectations about the problem(s).
- Carry out appropriate physical examination and near patient tests to confirm or refute the diagnosis.
- Reconsider your assessment of the problem.
- Reach a shared understanding of the problem with the patient.
- Give the patient advice about what they need to do to tackle the problem(s).
- Explain the action(s) you will be taking.
- Summarise and close.

This describes the sequence of events as they occur in a generic consultation. Although at first sight consultations involving children may seem very different to others, this outline actually remains a good order of events to have in your mind as you prepare for and go through the consultation. It is useful to fall back on if you become lost, bogged down or sidetracked. Read the model of the consultation above again, picturing a mother and child. The only adjustment needed is to replace the word 'patient' with 'child and mother' or 'child and family'.

In order for a consultation to go well, certain competencies are required by the health professional being consulted by the child and mother. The Consultation Assessment and Improvement Instrument for Nurses (CAIIN) describes them.[6] Although written for nurses undertaking new roles as independent prescribers, the CAIIN offers generic competencies and is based on similar models for GPs and medical students.[7] One example has been used to test medical students and doctors working with children, but it can also be applied to anyone performing a consultation involving children.[8]

Consultation competencies for children and families

Interviewing	Puts children and parents at ease
	Enables children and parents to explain situation(s)/problem(s) fully
	Listens attentively
	Seeks clarification of words used by children and parents as appropriate
	Demonstrates an ability to formulate open questions
	Phrases questions simply and clearly
	Uses silence appropriately
	Recognises children and parents' verbal and non-verbal cues
	Considers physical, social and psychological factors as appropriate
	Demonstrates a well-organised approach to information gathering
Examination, diagnostic tests and practical procedures	Elicits physical signs correctly and sensitively
	Uses instruments in a competent and sensitive manner
	Performs technical procedures in a competent and sensitive manner
Care planning and patient management	Formulates and follows appropriate care plans
	Reaches a shared understanding about the problem with children and parents
	Negotiates care plans with children and parents
	Uses clear and understandable language
	Educates children and parents appropriately in practical procedures
	Makes discriminating use of referral, investigation and drug treatment
	Arranges appropriate follow-up
Problem solving	Accesses relevant information from children and parents' records
	Explores children and parents' ideas, concerns and expectations about their problem(s)
	Elicits relevant information from children and parents
	Seeks relevant clinical signs and makes appropriate use of clinical tests
	Correctly interprets information gathered
	Applies clinical knowledge appropriately in the identification and management of the children and parents' problem(s)
	Recognises limits of personal competence and acts accordingly
Behaviour and relationship with children and parents	Maintains friendly but professional relationship with children and parents
	Conveys sensitivity to the needs of children and parents
	Is able to use the professional relationship in a manner likely to achieve mutual agreement on the care plan
Health promotion and disease prevention	Acts on appropriate opportunities for health promotion and disease prevention
	Provides appropriate explanation to children and parents for preventive initiatives suggested
	Works in partnership with children and parents to encourage the adoption of a healthier lifestyle

(continued)

Record keeping	Makes an appropriate and legible record of the consultation
	Records care plan to include advice and follow-up arrangements as appropriate
	Enters results of measurements in records
	Provides the name(s), dose and quantity of drug(s) prescribed together with any special precautions

We shall go through a consultation from the start, making reference to the model of the consultation and consultation competencies as we consider how to involve and communicate effectively with children and families.

Before you begin:

1. Interpret prior knowledge
   You will probably already have access to some information about this family. It is worth refreshing your memory before you start.
   — Family and social background: think about this particular family – who lives in the family home? What is their social and cultural background? Are they well known to you or your colleagues? Is English their first language?
   — Age and developmental stage of the child: you will need to know about this child's cognitive and physical development. Are they at the level expected for their age, or falling behind? How will you speak and communicate with this particular child?
   — Likely expectations of the child and family: what do both the child and parent expect to happen? Is this a new problem or a follow-up visit?

2. Set goals
   — Think about what you would ideally like to happen.
   — Is the aim the correct diagnosis of a medical problem, and agreement about its management?
   — Is this a routine health encounter (e.g. immunisation) but with health promotion possibilities? This may be a family who will not seek medical attention other than for routine health visits. Is this therefore one of the few opportunities to influence the family, or could this be used as a health promotion opportunity?
   — Is this a follow-up visit to confirm an agreed management plan is being maintained? Is the aim therefore just to reinforce an agreed plan and confirm that it is working for this family?

3. Think about how to put the child and carer at ease
   — There are a number of things you can do before meeting the family to facilitate the ease of both the child and the parent. How the room is laid out is important: where will we all sit? Are there enough chairs? How will the child or any siblings be occupied during the times that I need to talk to Mum? Are there any quiet toys to put out for a younger child or to put away for a teenager?
   — Environment also matters: for young babies especially the room should not

be too hot or cold. Whatever the age of the child, the room needs to feel neither too formal nor too 'clinical'.

4. Be aware of your ideas and theirs
    — The child and family: the mother and most children may have perceptions of you based on your role and their impressions of you from any previous meetings. If they have met you before – did it go well? If not, how will you do things differently this time? If they haven't met you, do they know who you are or what your role is? Have they had much contact with medical professionals in the past?
    — You: consciously review your perceptions of the child and family – be careful not to prejudge or make assumptions. You will have ideas about your role – what are your expectations about what you can and should achieve? Will your ideas fit with theirs? We all come to consultations with our family background as 'baggage' and will also have ideas about what constitutes a family. These ideas can be deep-rooted, but your ideas about what is acceptable or normal will inevitably be very different to those of other people.

5. Think about non-verbal communication
    — Even young children and babies respond to your non-verbal signals, so be very conscious of what messages you are sending. We can use non-verbal communication to facilitate information gathering so be as deliberate in this as you are in your verbal communication. Equally, be alert to the non-verbal messages of everyone in the room – parents, child siblings or grandparents. While listening to one person, prepare to be watching all the others so as not to miss any non-verbal cues.

Introductions

First impressions count so take special care with introductions. The only one in the room whose name you know is likely to be the child's, whose name you called (and occasionally not even that if you or they are not paying attention!). Find a sensitive way to check who the adults are – they may not be Mum and Dad. We all occasionally forget this golden rule, but there is nothing like addressing an older Mum as 'Granny' to put you in your place!

With families I don't know I always check:

➤ With a baby or young child: 'So this is Jane . . .?' Wait for confirmation. Then ask the adult, 'And you are . . .?'
➤ With an older child: 'So you are Jane . . .?' Wait for confirmation. 'And who have you brought with you . . .?' or, 'And who's this?'

With older children check also what they like to be called – Chris may only be Christopher when he has done something wrong; using his full name may make him think he's in trouble. Michael may hate that everyone assumes he prefers Mike, so using the abbreviation may reduce his cooperation with you.

Having established who they are, you then need to introduce yourself to parent and child, using appropriately straightforward and jargon-free language. Tell them your name, deciding whether you will use your first name or your surname, together with a title: 'I am Mary, a children's nurse' or, 'I'm Dr Patel, a children's doctor'. Also tell them what is going to happen in the consultation. Children can be very worried about the unknown; if you can explain and reassure, this will relax them and they will be more likely to participate. For instance, if a child had a blood test on a previous visit and you know that one is not needed this time say so very early on.

Making the introductions is a good way to try to engage the child right from the start. Most children of playgroup age and above can tell you their name and age.

CASE SCENARIO 1

Starting the consultation

You call Alisa, a two-year-old girl. She goes to Mum who holds her hand on the way to your room. Dad follows. They chat in a language you later discover is Ukrainian. On entering the room Alisa sits on Mum's lap, with Dad in the other chair. Dad does not speak English so Mum does the talking after chatting sometimes with Dad.

A few minutes later Mum stops. You notice an ID badge round her neck. 'You do realise, don't you, that I'm the interpreter . . .?'

'I'm sorry, it's just that Alisa obviously knows you well. I had assumed you were Mum . . .'

'The Ukrainian community is very small here – I am a close family friend as well.'

Interviewing and information gathering

Establish who will be telling the story – this depends on the age, developmental stage and to some extent the personality of child and their wishes.

Younger children may well not do much more than give their name and age early on, as they need to understand that Mum thinks of you as friendly before they will trust you enough to speak – offer them a quiet toy, a book or paper and pencil. Watch them and wait for their non-verbal cues that they are ready to talk. Be aware of the need for multitasking with toddlers. A mother may be holding two conversations at once – one with you and another with the child. This can be confusing if you are not used to it, but parents are very skilled at this – it gets easier with practice.

Older children, even teenagers, will often defer to Mum given the choice. You will need to respect this but also try to keep them involved and engaged. Don't give up on getting them involved – it is worth it in the longer term. Try non-controversial topics first as sometimes after one or two sentences a child's confidence will grow.

When you ask a question to a child, you will need to be patient as they will often take longer to formulate a reply – use their name and keep eye contact with them; if you look at mother she will take over and your chance to get the child's view will be lost.

There will be times when you need to get the views of the mother, or information that the child is unable or unwilling to give. At these times, remember that children are listening even when they look like they are not – once you start a conversation with the mother it is easier than you think to forget the presence of the child and say something inappropriate.

There are a few other general points to consider in your information gathering with families.

➤ Use of language: in all consultations you need to watch for jargon but this is especially true when talking with children. This will require you to simplify things for younger children and to find out the words they use for certain things, such as body parts and functions.

➤ Verbal and non-verbal cues: we have already mentioned the importance of noticing non-verbal cues, but also listen for verbal cues from all in the room. The muttered comment from a teenager may give the biggest clue as to what is going on and the interruption from Granny may help you to understand family dynamics.

➤ Family and social background: you will have considered this before you start and you may know this family well, but if not you can get a lot of information as you observe how they talk and interact with you and each other.

➤ Different versions of events: in getting children to tell their own story, we will run into times when their answers disagree with the mother's. This needs to be handled sensitively. Younger children may misremember or give what they think is the 'right answer'. All children may wish to avoid unpleasant things like tests or medicines and answer accordingly. This all needs to be taken into account when clarifying exactly what has happened.

CASE SCENARIO 2

A challenge to involving a child

Mary is 11. She has come with headaches. There are no worrying features in the history, but Mum is very anxious. Mary says nothing, so Mum is doing all the talking. You notice Mary's body language and feel that she does not agree with Mum's version of events.

- How will you try to engage her in conversation?
- How will you encourage Mum to let her daughter give her version of events?
- How will you handle any disagreement?

Ideas, concerns and expectations

The ideas, concerns and expectations of both the parents and the child need to be considered – it is surprisingly easy to assume that the child has no ideas, concerns or expectations, but they often do. Think about how you can ask children what they think is wrong, what their worries are and what they would like you to do. They may well not be able to articulate all of these to you, but it is worth trying, and is sometimes very revealing.

Examination

Depending on the reason for the encounter, there may not be much need for examination, but we will take the consultation to find a diagnosis and make a plan of management as our example for now.

By the end of the history, you should know the most likely diagnosis. A targeted examination to look for particular signs is then used to confirm this or to exclude other possible diagnoses.

Remember that children may even dislike what we would think of as a simple and painless examination.

Often, especially with young children and infants, you will need to be opportunistic, not necessarily sticking to a rigid routine. Provided you complete all relevant examinations it doesn't matter what order you do it in, or indeed where you do it. Don't move a young child until you have to – sitting on Mum's lap is just fine for most examinations. If Mum is cuddling the infant with his back to you, you may well be able to listen to the back of a fractious child's chest before he notices and cries. Distraction is also a useful technique for younger infants – use a quiet toy of theirs or yours to keep their attention and they may not grab and eat your stethoscope.

For slightly older children, make it a game. For example, for abdominal examination, 'I bet I can guess what you had for breakfast. It will be in here, won't it? I think you had . . .' The central nervous system examination can also easily be turned into a game, especially if you join in: 'Can you walk like you're on a tightrope like me?' and, 'I want to see if you are stronger than me'.

Be sensitive to teenagers – uncover them as little as possible, ask them who they would like present, and have as few in the room as possible. Chaperoning needs to be mentioned here. It is obviously important not to examine a teenager without someone else in the room to act as a chaperone.

At the end of any examination, reconsider your assessment. Are you now sure of a diagnosis? Can you move on to a negotiated management plan or are any tests needed?

Tests and procedures

Sometimes a practical procedure is the reason for a health encounter (e.g. vaccination). In this case clearly the procedure is necessary. In other cases it may not be.

Think – is this really needed?

If it is:

➤ always explain before doing, but not using scary words
➤ never pretend it won't hurt if it will
➤ let the parent be there, and try to make them the good guy
➤ the professional and parents should encourage the child to cope[9]
➤ be as quick, competent and kind as possible
➤ actively involve children in distraction techniques both during and after the procedure.[9]

Management

In order to form a management plan, you need to reach a shared understanding of the problem(s) with the parents and child. This shared understanding is more than just giving a correct diagnosis – a better approach is to create a problem list. Having done this, your management plan should then include agreeing on a solution for each identified problem together with the parents and child.

CASE SCENARIO 3

Compiling the problem list

A young first-time Mum with no support network brings her four-month-old, Anna, to see you. Anna is well in herself, but had diarrhoea and vomiting for 24 hours.

What could be the possible problem list? Think of the three categories in the biopsychosocial model of disease.

In this case scenario just to say your baby has gastroenteritis will not really help this mother and baby. There may be medical (dehydration and a sore bottom), psychological (guilt about not sterilising the bottle correctly; maternal isolation) and social (having to take time off work; looking after other children) problems to consider. If you are faced with a child with a number of problems, you may need to choose just one or two to start with and come back to the others.

Reaching a shared understanding can be a challenge, even more so in dealing with children as this understanding needs to be formed with several parties. With older children start by addressing the child in simple terms to see if they can grasp the problem and potential solutions. If successful, this involvement can improve health outcomes. It has the added advantage that the parent is listening and so may not need much more information. With younger children the emphasis moves to the parent, but the child is likely to be listening so be wary about what you say.

What about when parents and child disagree? The views of a teenager who is 'Gillick competent' (*see* Chapter 8 for more detail) generally take precedence over those of a parent, as to do otherwise would be in breach of the ethical principle of autonomy. But what about a six-year-old who refuses to let you examine his throat? The young child has a right to have their views heard but any consent required is from the parent. If the parent agrees with the need to examine then it can go ahead. It is good to try to help a young child to see why a medicine or procedure, etc., is needed, but beware asking for their permission – how will you handle the answer, 'No!'? Rather than ask for their consent to something you will have to do anyway, offer them a limited choice. 'I need to look at your tummy – do you want to stay on Mum's lap or climb onto our big bed?'

What about when the parents disagree with each other? Fortunately this is rare and with sensitive perseverance it can usually be resolved. Often you hear about disagreement only from the one parent who is accompanying the child. There may, however, be times when you need to be clear about who has parental responsibility and who has custody of the child.

Written explanation

It is usually a good idea to back up what has been said with written information. Both children and adults often respond well to, and remember better, a drawing or diagram as part of an explanation.

If you don't feel comfortable about your artistic abilities, then it is good to make use of information leaflets written for both parents and children. These may exist in your place of work. If not it is worth finding out what exists on the Internet or from patient support groups. There are good and bad Internet sites and a lot of parents and teenagers will look things up, so why not give them the web addresses of a couple of good sites that you have already pre-checked and know are a reliable source of information?

The national guidance is to copy patients into any correspondence and many doctors already do this. It is always worth considering writing to parents after the consultation, to reinforce what was said. There can be a large disagreement between professionals and patients about what was said in a consultation and a letter can help to clarify things.[10]

Ending the consultation

This is not always as easy as it seems, and some families and patients can appear to be extremely reluctant to leave. This may be because we have not addressed all the issues they have come with, or because we have not really reached a shared understanding.

We all have deadlines and must try to keep to time if we can. If we let this consultation drag on, the next will be harder. On the other hand there are some conversations that can't easily be cut short. Signposting the order of events at the start and at intervals as the consultation proceeds helps families to know where they are in the process and to know when it is time to go. In explaining this to the child in very straightforward terms, we know that the parent is also listening. Remember that families may also have deadlines – it is courteous to check, especially if they were called in late. If it is clear the parent would continue for a lot longer than you have time for, explain time is up and arrange a follow-up for further discussion if necessary.

CONCLUSION

It is very important to engage with children in the consultation process. In using these techniques to facilitate involvement of children in the consultation we will remind the families and ourselves that it is the child who is our patient. Furthermore, we will have involved and less disruptive children, who cooperate more, are more engaged in their management plans and experience better outcomes.

REFERENCES

1 Cahill P, Papageorgiou A. Triadic communication in the primary care paediatric consultation: a review of the literature. *Brit J Gen Pract.* 2007; **57**: 904–11.

2 *Children Act 1989.* London: HMSO; 1989. c.41. Available at: www.opsi.gov.uk/acts/acts1989/ukpga_19890041_en_1 (accessed 14 June 2010).

3 British Medical Association (BMA). *Consent, Rights and Choices in Health Care for Children and Young People.* London: BMJ Books; 2001.

4 Department of Health. *National Service Framework for Children, Young People and Maternity Services.* London: DH Publications; 2004.

5 Lewis C, Rachelefsky G, Lewis M, *et al.* A randomized trial of A.C.T. (Asthma Care Training) for kids. *Pediatrics.* 1984; **74**: 478–86.

6 Hastings AM, Redsell SA (editors). *The Good Consultation Guide for Nurses.* Oxford: Radcliffe Medical Press; 2006.

7 McKinley RK, Fraser RC, Van der Vleuten C, *et al.* Formative assessment of the consultation performance of medical students in the setting of general practice using a modified version of the Leicester Assessment Package. *Med Educ.* 2000; **34**(7): 573–9.

8 Howells RJ, Davis H, Silverman J, *et al.* Assessment of doctors' consultation skills in the paediatric setting: the Paediatric Consultation Assessment Tool. *Arch Dis Child.* 2010 (2008); **95**(5): 323–9. Available at: http://adc.bmj.com/content/95/5/323.full (accessed 14 June 2010).

9 Cohen L. Behavioral approaches to anxiety and pain management for pediatric venous access. *Pediatrics.* 2008; **122**: S134–S139.

10 Parkin T, Skinner TC. Discrepancies between patient and professionals recall and perception of an outpatient consultation. *Diabetic Med.* 2003; **20**: 909–14.

CHAPTER 5

Professional speak and child talk

Elizabeth Anderson and Sarah Redsell

This chapter reviews the approaches taken to communicating with children and young people by a range of education, health and social care professionals. The chapter does not cover medical communication as this is covered elsewhere in this book (Chapters 3, 4 and 5). Evidence from a range of different disciplines will be outlined using the psychosocial development model of Erikson, so that the skills of a particular profession can be related to the developmental stage of the child.[1] The chapter takes a primary care perspective and considers the following disciplines:

➤ nursing: midwife, health visitor, school nurse and practice nurse
➤ nursery nurse
➤ speech and language therapy
➤ social work
➤ school counsellor
➤ teacher.

These insights will provide tips for improving communication with children and young people, illustrated through case examples and vignettes. The development of communication skills for working with children will be related to each profession. Consideration will be given to curriculum directives and how these are translated into training. The chapter proceeds to discuss how the professions who work with children now form the Children's Workforce and are required to work together in responding to child and family needs.[2,3] This requires preparation for team working in which each of the different professional perspectives are understood; shared and effective interprofessional communication becomes the norm.

INTRODUCTION

Children and young people's health and well-being is the domain of many disciplines from those who work within the social spectrum (e.g. social workers and youth workers) to those who work within the health spectrum (e.g. therapists and nurses).

In general, the majority of healthy children and young people only access universal services, which include early years practitioners (child minders, playgroup workers, crèche workers, nursery nurses and child-centre staff); school staff (teachers, special education needs coordinators and classroom assistants); and health professionals (midwives, health visitors, general practitioners (GPs), practice nurses and school health nurses/advisors). Some children and young people require additional targeted specialist provision, including speech and language therapists (S and LTs), specialist teachers and health visitors, educational psychologists, occupational therapists, physiotherapists, counsellors, paediatricians and hospital specialists.

Each professional discipline approaches communication with children and young people from a different perspective (*see* Table 5.1). This is based upon the context within which they encounter children and young people; for example, some professions work with children at home, in school, playgroup, nursery or community settings. Others encounter sick children and young people in clinics, emergency rooms and hospital wards. These different insights are extremely helpful when faced with challenging and complex situations validating the need for interprofessional working. An analysis of each discipline's professional standards exposes large differences in emphasis for curriculum content of communication-skills training (*see* Table 5.2). In general, little curriculum time focuses on the skill of communicating with children and young people and the expectation is that these skills will be learnt in practice, supported by practitioners who act as clinical tutors or mentors. However, the Social Care Institute for Excellence (SCIE) recently commissioned a review of the teaching, learning and assessment of communication skills with children for social work training.[4] This review highlights the problem of teaching specialist skills, such as communication with children, on generic courses and the lack of clarity about the range and level of skill taught. It acknowledges that there is a lack of consensus about what 'makes communication skilled' (p. 12) and emphasises the challenge of involving patients and members of the public in professional training (which poses ethical problems, as children are mostly excluded), leaving much learning to be completed through practice supervision and instruction.[5,6] Lefevre and colleagues outline a taxonomy of core skills and conditions for the qualifying level curriculum for social work.[7] However, in contrast, there is little curriculum content devoted to communication skill development for health visitors and the emphasis is on public health and needs assessment skills. Public health nurses choosing children and families registration are expected to develop communication skills while in practice.[8]

In gathering data for this chapter, time has been spent listening afresh to colleagues' reflections on their work and interactions with children. Most of their skills are drawn from experience and nothing will replace the opportunity to engage with as many children and young people as possible to realise the, sometimes impossible, task of understanding children's responses and reactions.[9] Many are working at the highest level of competence and speak about their innate ability to 'just know' and have that 'gut feeling'.[10]

TABLE 5.1 The roles and responsibilities of health and social care professionals working with children

Practitioner	Role	Responsibilities and reference to communication with children	Source of data
Professionals who all work with children			
Health visitor (Specialist public health nurses with child and young families)	Work within primary healthcare team and the wider community on health promotion and prevention. Unique one-to-one relationship with families of pre-school children. Work is underpinned by four public health domains: • search for health needs • stimulation of awareness of health needs • influence on policies affecting health • facilitation of health-enhancing activities.	Child emotional and physical development, especially attainment of key milestones. Expertise in public health and family support. They have core competencies in working with vulnerable children and young people including child protection. They require effective communication with children and young people and child development and behaviours (page 7). In relation to communication the recent publication by the chief nursing officer added their need for skills in mental health, listening and communication with children. Also support for fathers and families of children with physical and learning disabilities and leading skill-mixed teams (page 8).	Nursing and Midwifery Council. Standards of proficiency for specialist community public health nurses. The Chief Nursing officer's review of the nursing, midwifery and health visiting contribution to vulnerable children and young people. Department of Health (2004), London.
School nurse	School nurses work with all school-aged children and young people, especially those who are vulnerable. They assess health needs and engage in immunisation and preventative health strategies in schools.	In relation to communication the chief nursing officer states it remains essential that Children's Trusts and PCTs and local authorities ensure access to their services for first contact and acute care, long-term conditions and public health for school-aged children.	Nursing and Midwifery Council. Standards of proficiency for specialist community public health nurses.

(continued)

Practitioner	Role	Responsibilities and reference to communication with children	Source of data
School nurse (*cont.*)	Work within schools under the umbrella of the specialist community and public health nurses following the four domains as outlined for health visiting.	School nurses are required to lead and or work in skill-mixed teams with youth workers, health-advisers, young people and teachers, social workers and others.	The Chief Nursing Officer's review of the nursing, midwifery and health visiting contribution to vulnerable children and young people. Department of Health (2004), London.
Midwife	A practising midwife ensures care of a woman and baby during the antenatal, intranatal and postnatal period (NMC 2004; 16 Rule 6).	Communicate effectively with women and their families throughout the pre-conception, antenatal, intrapartum and the postnatal period (page 21). The chief nursing officer states midwives should be integral to the work of children's centres and work within skill-mixed teams using maternity care assessments. Midwives offer ongoing continuity of care working with health visitors and PHCTs to ensure flexible ongoing support following birth.	The Nursing and Midwifery Council. The Chief Nursing Officer's review of the nursing, midwifery and health visiting contribution to vulnerable children and young people. Department of Health (2004), London.
Nursery nurse	Early Years, or nursery, teachers work in pre-school, nursery and reception classes with children aged between three and five.	This involves motivating children to learn and imaginatively using resources in order to facilitate learning.	In England, Wales and Northern Ireland, the main qualification is the National Nursery Examination Board (NNEB) Diploma in Nursery Nursing (two years, full-time, also available part-time), awarded by the Council for Awards in Children's Care and Education (CACHE). In Scotland, the most common route is to take a National Certificate or National Qualification course, which lasts one year.

Practitioner	Role	Responsibilities and reference to communication with children	Source of data
Nursery nurse (*cont.*)			Children's Workforce Development Council (CWDC). Sector for Skills Council and Skills for Care and Development. (www.cwdcouncil.org.uk) National Day Nurseries Association (www.ndna.org.uk) Early Years workforce: National Early Years Enterprise Centre.
Teacher	Maximise children and young people's ability to learn and develop. Their main role is in developing people and improving young lives.	Qualified teachers [Qualified Teacher Status (QTS)] must work towards expecting high expectations of children and young people including a commitment to ensuring that they can achieve their full educational potential. This depends upon communication that is established on a fair, respectful, trusting, supportive and constructive relationship. Communicating and working with others is an essential responsibility.	Award of qualified teacher status is given by the General Teaching Council for England following accreditation by the Initial Teacher Training (ITT) provider on assessment of the Quality Teaching Standards (QTS). Training and Development Agency (TDA), 2007.

Professionals who work with children who require specialist help and or support

Community paediatrician	Responsibilities for the care of children outside of hospital.	Locality assessment and management of general paediatric problems and chronic illness in a variety of non-hospital settings.	General Medical Council. Royal College of Paediatrics and Child Health.

(*continued*)

Practitioner	Role	Responsibilities and reference to communication with children	Source of data
Community paediatrician *(cont.)*	Specialist diagnostic work with skills and expertise in child development, immunisation, and educational and social needs for children with disabilities or special needs.	Child public health and population paediatrics including immunisation. Assessment and management of behavioural and development problems, neuro-disability and multi-agency assessment. Social paediatrics and child protection clinical assessment. Level 1 has 13 competences for communication with children and young people (page 20) which includes; skills and strategies to manage consultations effectively with babies, young children, adolescents and their families; skills to involve both the child and parents or carers when both are present in consultations.	A Framework of Competences for Level 1 training in Paediatrics, Royal College of Paediatrics and Child Health (June 2008).
Social worker	Work with individuals, families, carers, groups and communities to assess their needs and circumstances to promote personal development and empowerment. Social work intervenes at the points where people interact with their environments.	Their assessment responsibilities are for the individual and/or family, carer, and for groups and communities in relationship to needs and circumstances. In this role they have responsibilities to advocate for others and represent their needs, views and circumstances. They manage risk and carry out the statutory duties of the authority; for example, in looking after children and young people which might involve placing them for adoption or foster care.	General Social Care Council. International Association of Schools of Social Work and the International Federation of Social Workers.

Practitioner	Role	Responsibilities and reference to communication with children	Source of data
Speech and language therapist	Therapists work with children and young people to assess communication and developmental needs. They will provide an evidence-based service that anticipates and responds to the needs of the individuals who experience speech, language, communication or swallowing difficulties.	Assess children's communication and identify and put into place a therapeutic management plan. Preventative work focusing on children or communities at risk. Partnership work with families to ensure holistic approach and the ability to share skills with other professionals, training teachers and healthcare workers. Key to their success is the development of a therapeutic relationship with the child and family. The relationship must be built on trust and empathy.	Health Professions Council. Royal College of Speech and Language Therapists.

TABLE 5.2 Generic competency and standards for practitioners who communicate with children and young people

Profession	Professional body*	Accountability/Standard description
Health visitor	Nursing and Midwifery Council. *Standards and Proficiency for Specialist Community Public Health Nurses.* (www.nmc-uk.org)	Public Health Nursing. Principle: Surveillance and assessment of the population's health and well-being. • Develop and sustain relationships with groups and individuals with the aim of improving health and social well-being.
Midwife	Royal College of Midwives. Nursing and midwifery Council (www.nmc-uk.org)	Essential Skills Clusters 1. Communication *Be attentive and share information that is clear, accurate and meaningful at a level which women, their partners and family can understand*
Nursery nurse	Children Workforce Development Council (CWDC). Sector for Skills Council and Skills for Care and Development (www.cwdcouncil.org.uk) National Day Nurseries Association (www.ndna.org.uk) Early Years workforce: National Early Years Enterprise Centre	Level 3: Integrated Qualifications Framework The Department for Children, Schools and Families 2008 stated in its document entitled *2020 Children and Young People's Workforce Strategy*[46] that by 2011 the NVQ Level 3 qualification for play workers who may be named 'Early Years professionals' would be outlined. At the moment training varies although experience in the nursery setting where communication skills are taught remains a key area for skills development.
Paediatrician	Royal College of Paediatrics and Child Health. (www.rcpch.ac.uk/)	Level 1: Communication skills in paediatrics (n=13), *three examples* • Understand the need to conduct a consultation in such a way that a child or young person and their family feel able to talk about difficult emotional issues • Show patience and sensitivity in their communication with children and their families and a particular ability to explore their individual perspectives of a problem. • Have begun to develop active listening skills with children and young people and understand the need to respect their views in accordance with their age, maturity.

Profession	Professional body*	Accountability/Standard description
Speech and language therapist	Standards of Proficiency: Health Professions Council (www.hpc-uk.org) Royal College of Speech and Language Therapists (www.rcslt.org)	1.b.3: be able to demonstrate effective and appropriate skills in communication *(extracts only)* • Understand how communication skills affect the assessment of service users . . . modify for . . . age. • Be able to select, move between and use appropriate forms of verbal and non-verbal communication. • Be aware of the characteristics and consequences of non-verbal communication. • Provide service users with the information necessary to enable them to make informed decisions. • Recognise that relationships with service users should be based on mutual respect and trust. 1.b.4: understand the need for effective communication throughout the care of the service users.
Social worker	Department of Health (www.doh.gov.uk) General Social Care Council (www.gscc.org.uk) National Occupancy Standards for Social Work	Requirements for Social Work Training Providers will have to ensure students undertake specific learning and assessment in the following key areas: • communication skills with children, adults and those with particular communication needs. Key Role 1: • work with individuals, families, carers, groups and communities to help them to make informed decisions • assess needs and option to recommend a course of action.
Teacher	Professional Standards for Teachers in England 2007 Training and Development Agency for Schools (TDA) (www.tda.gov.uk) QTS: Qualifying to Teach (www.teach-tta.gov.uk)	*Standards for Qualified Teacher Status:* Relationships with children and young people: Q1. *Have high expectations of children and young people including a commitment to ensuring that they can achieve their full educational potential and to establishing fair, respectful, trusting, supportive and constructive relationships with them.* Communicating and working with others: Q4. *Communicate effectively with children, young people, colleagues, parents and carers.* Outcome statements to be met at the end of training. Documented as a portfolio of evidence.

* *Methods of assessing communication skills vary across each discipline according to their standards and competencies. In many cases standards of competency are not stated in the curriculum.*

Competence learning model

- Unconscious incompetence: the person is not aware of the existence or relevance of the skill area. The person does not know what s/he does not know. The learner is in a state of 'blissful ignorance'. Confidence exceeds ability.
- Conscious incompetence: the person becomes aware of the existence and relevance of the skills and also aware of their deficiency in this area. Confidence reduces with the realisation that ability is limited. Practice is essential for learning.
- Conscious competence: the person achieves conscious competence in a skill when they can perform it reliably at will. The person needs to concentrate and think in order to perform the skills.
- Unconscious competence: the person can perform the skill but does not necessarily know how s/he does it – it becomes second nature.

Children and young people's communication needs differ according to their age, cognitive development and social context (*see* Chapter 2). This chapter will explore professional communication at each of the psychosocial development or life stages of Erikson's framework[1] outlined below:

'INFANT' 0–1½ years = Trust versus Mistrust. A focus on the relationship with the mother and oral exploration of the world.

'TODDLER' 1–3 years = Autonomy versus Shame and doubt. A focus on learning bodily control through toilet training and the pleasure of pleasing parents.

'PRESCHOOL' 3–6 years = Initiative versus Guilt. A focus on sexual identity and awareness of birth and origins.

'SCHOOL-AGE' 6–12 years = Industry versus Inferiority. A focus on learning.

'ADOLESCENT' 12–18 years = Identity versus Role confusion. A focus on puberty and its associated body changes.

INFANT (0–1½) = TRUST VERSUS MISTRUST

The midwife and the health visitor team

Midwives and health visitors work with all families, the former predominantly in communication with the parents of a newborn infant and the latter through several child developmental stages in prior to school entry (*see* Table 5.1). Over the first six months of life the infant emerges as a social human being and learns to exchange signals and to communicate with their primary caregiver.[11] Health professionals are highly skilled guests during this phase and can help initiate and also pick up on these communication signals alerting colleagues such as the GP if they identify problems requiring further investigation.

The mother's repertoire of signal-giving to an infant indicates the development of a bond which normally comes naturally between infant and mother,[12] then father and extended family members. These exchanges involve a full range of emotional facial displays combined with vocalisations. The mother's gentle tones and voice oscillations are accompanied by the infant's gurgles and range of noises.

These early interactions are important but a mother's responsiveness to her infant can be affected by a number of factors including premature birth, trauma at birth, the unexpected birth of a disabled child, post-natal depression and infant temperament.[13] Lack of early emotional attachments can be a warning for health professionals as evidence of failure to bond with the infant.[14,15] Health professionals who visit and observe mother–infant interactions at around the tenth day post-natally refer to this period of communication as 'getting in tune'. Attachment screening tools are available.[16] Murray and Andrews have captured these communications in photograph action strips in *The Social Baby*.[17]

Communicating with baby

Movement of eyes, mouth, eyebrows and facial muscles display: joy, surprise, fear, anger, disgust, sadness.

Example: wide eyes (e.g. eyebrow raising or flashing to indicate surprise, flirting, greeting) show a readiness to interact, as opposed to narrow eyes (knitted eyebrows in anger, fear, disapproval), which imply a reduced readiness for interaction.

TOP TIP

Get close and personal with the baby – all these conversations are designed to take place at the distance from mother's face to the breast.

Gentle tones and soft speaking as reflected by mother (men should be aware they may need to modulate their voice).

TODDLER (1–3 YEARS) = AUTONOMY VERSUS SHAME AND DOUBT
The health visiting team

Rapid changes take place physically, mentally and socially within the first years of an infant's life and health professionals' communication strategies need to adapt accordingly. In particular, the beginnings of independence are visible in toddlers' behaviour patterns and communication depends upon understanding how they see the world. The family unit plays a significant part in how the child develops communication strategies and error can lead to behavioural frustrations. Health professionals need to recognise that a toddler learns through repetition, following and modelling others' behaviours. Health professionals develop skills to communicate with the toddlers by literally getting into the child's world by adjusting to their height level, using words that clearly refer to what they mean, losing any self-consciousness to enter their imagination and play along with them. Communication is best achieved with the comfort of familiarity and a carer's presence is often helpful as toddlers are fearful of strangers. Toddlers' worlds are limited and there may be cultural differences in the use and meaning of words.[18] Meaning will not necessarily align to adult use; for example, 'no' may mean 'yes'. There are some excellent resources with examples of behaviours at this stage shown pictorially and demonstrated with everyday situations in *The Social Toddler*.[19] The box below offers 'top tips' for communicating with toddlers, where professionals must remember that the toddler 'knows if you are really interested in them'.

Communicating with toddlers

Example: Let the toddler observe you before you observe them. Avert your gaze onto a toy or some activity until they appear relaxed and not threatened by you. Approach the child by getting down to their level and through play. Speak quietly and with confidence; ask them, 'Can I look at your doll/car?', and when in their circle of trust offer face and eye contact and smile.

TOP TIPS

AVOID:
- bombarding the child with questions
- overreacting to negative behaviour – turn away and make no response.

MUST DO:
- offer age-appropriate toys
- talk simply at their level of comprehension; consider *tone*, *voice*, *pace* and *volume*
- draw pictures; engage in a distracting set of play activities
- quickly become familiar with their 'world' (e.g. 'In my night garden . . .')
- show interest in what they are saying and believe in this; engage in communication using open eye gestures, confirmatory words (e.g. 'yes',' OK')
- use bite-size chunks of words
- always get down to their level
- know when to avoid eye contact (always on first meeting until you know they have taken in you and your surroundings)
- take time before getting physically close and before interaction
- make sure they are the centre of your attention
- consider your physical facial expressions – be smiling
- praise good behaviour
- where possible sit and share a book together.

Toddlers display emotions that reveal insights into their social world and are expressed through behaviour. Health professionals have a list of behaviours they look for when working with a child, which can indicate concerns for either physical or emotional care.

Children vary in their cognitive development at this age and there is a gap between what they can understand and what they can articulate. Some of the work which has highlighted this comes from studies exploring children's reaction to bereavement.[20,21] This has shown that professionals need to consider associations and timing of conversations and remember that toddlers' comprehension may exceed their ability to express what they understand verbally. For example, when explaining to a toddler that a member of the family has died, using the colloquial phrase, 'we've lost your sister', may not be appropriate. This will challenge their knowledge and experience of English, and the child may respond, 'let's go and find her then'. During this phase children are egocentric and view themselves as central to the universe. In any dialogue with a child health professionals need to speak directly and try not to use abstract concepts or metaphors.

Behaviour: concerns

Be ALERT to:
- evading all eye contact
- flinching near to parent
- clinging onto professionals
- abnormally tearful
- what is not appropriate for their age (e.g. sexual understanding of body changes)
- a child who repeatedly fails to attend appointments, or has an increase in A&E visits
- be aware of all non-verbal clues (e.g. itching, a child who keeps checking parent with quick glances)
- disclosures (e.g. 'Can I tell you what happened to Mummy', etc.).

The nursery nurse

Nursery nurses communicate with infants and children using play to design learning for the foundation or pre-school period of child development (*see* Table 5.1). As previously outlined, toddlers like to be near those they feel familiar with and preferably to have their mother nearby. Attending local nurseries and playgroups can be very challenging, and normally children are distressed if and when their mother leaves. Communicating with toddlers about parents leaving and returning requires special skills. These moments need clear explanation which is consistent between mother and carer. The carer then needs to take on the familiar person role during mother's absence. At the Baby and Toddler Nest (Pen Green Centre*) the nursery nurses spend a lot of time thinking about and supporting children with the separations and reunions from their parents and carers. They ensure they are available to warmly greet the children and chat to the parents. They talk to the parents about how they think their child will cope with being separated from them. This gives them an insight into the support the child may need. The nursery nurses also talk to the parents about how they would like their child to be supported through these experiences. They then closely observe the children as they separate from the parent and offer appropriate

---

* Pen Green Centre: www.pengreen.org/pengreencenter.php. *See* Acknowledgements (p. 82).

comfort and support to help them settle. Workers also tune in to children's reunions when their parents return to collect them. Once again, observing and supporting the child and the parent as they reunite after their absence from each other. At all times when the children are in the Baby and Toddler Nest, the nursery nurses will closely observe them and tune into their emotional well-being, offering comfort and support as the children need it. Here is an example of a child communicating and how workers responded.

An angry child

A child was extremely angry on separation from her parent. She shouted at the children and workers nearby. The nursery nurse tried to approach her and she pointed her finger, shouting, 'No'. The child moved away from the nursery nurse and other children and climbed behind the rocking chair and continued to shout at the other children and nursery nurse. She started to cry and shout loudly, pushing the rocking chair and kicking toys. The nursery nurse went over and sat close by, gently talking to her, saying to the child that she could see how angry she was. The child continued to cry and shout. The nursery nurse attempted to reach out to her, stretching her arm to stroke the child's back, but the child arched away. The nursery nurse explained that her Mummy had gone but she always came back. The child continued to shout and push the rocking chair. The worker continued to sit nearby quietly talking to the child, staying next to her, allowing her to show her feelings. In time the child was able to calm and the nursery nurse was able to approach her, pick her up and comfort her with a cuddle.

PRE-SCHOOL (3–6 years) = Initiative versus Guilt

The speech and language therapist

Speech and language therapists (S and LTs) work with children and young people identified as requiring targeted specialist provision (*see* Table 5.1). S and LTs endorse the belief that developing skills to communicate with children takes time, experience and reflection, and they also consider an ability to 'tune in' as vital. Effective communication with children is not, they perceive, about talking all of the time, asking lots of questions (to which we already know the answer!) or being the entertainer. Effective communication takes time to build and involves active listening and following the child's lead.

In 2003 the Royal College of Speech and Language Therapists launched I CAN, a comprehensive website containing information on all aspects of communication development, including up-to-date expert information for families and the children's workforce.[22] Some materials are books, such as 'talkabout', which is a useful guide to interact with children. Other material used by S and LTs is that of the Canadian Hanen programme. The Hanen Centre offers a range of resources for parents and professionals to improve children's communication. In particular, techniques in following a child's lead, observing, listening and waiting for children and methods of mapping to scaffold word development.

Speech and language therapists (S and LTs)

TOP TIPS

- Be aware of all aspects of language development and match your own language to the language level of the child. Keep language simple; use clear simple questions.
- Be aware that our understanding of language may vary from the child's and look for signs when communication has broken down. Often a child who does not understand will become distracted or answer a question incorrectly, in this case use visual support to supplement spoken language.
- Understand the importance and development of play so that interaction can take place through play.
- Hanen principles are useful. A training course to learn Hanen can be found at: www. hanen.org/web/Home/HealthcareProfessionals/tabid/58/Default.aspx.
- Be child-centred – understand and respect childhood culture. Tune in to the child's level and to 'see' things from a child's perspective.
- Following the child's pace of interaction (e.g. using pauses).

S and LTs learn techniques for interacting with children both in the classroom and experientially. They are perceived to be essential in overcoming the significant speech and language difficulties reported in a high number of children entering school. S and LTs can offer a child one-to-one therapy, providing techniques to develop relevant communication capacity. The recent Bercow Review highlighted the importance of the skills of this profession being cascaded to other professionals in the children's workforce, such as teachers and health visitors.[23]

CHILD (6–12 YRS) = INDUSTRY VERSUS INFERIORITY
The primary school teacher

A central task of teachers is to enable children to be better communicators. Like most professionals at this stage they need to know what is in the 'black box' and they work though assessments using formative and summative teaching methods (*see* Table 5.1). Frameworks for assessment of learning can help other disciplines working with children to understand the level of knowledge they can comprehend. Teachers spend many hours with young people and are in tune to communication expressed through behaviour. During this developmental phase children have the tendency to see themselves as central to what happens; this is known as 'centralising'.

A few children have communication needs that require additional support both from within and outside school. This may arise because they have special educational needs or because English is not their first language. Chapter 10 provides detailed advice about how individual professionals might approach communication with children with different types of special needs. Children with special educational needs usually have a host of professionals involved in their welfare. This might include social workers, who represent both the child and the parent, and health professionals looking after a specific need, for example occupational therapists to help with motor-coordination problems. The communication requirements of children with special educational needs are usually managed within schools by the special educational needs coordinator (SENCO). SENCOs are also involved in collecting the evidence for statutory assessment for those children who have significant needs beyond the school's provision. SENCOs also hold review meetings and ensure that all professionals involved in a child's welfare (class teachers, parents, outside agencies, learning support assistants and the child, as appropriate) contribute.

Teacher observation on centralising

Example: Children at this age consider themselves as central in the universe. In one teacher's experience a child became convinced she caused her father to die because the mother had asked her to 'be quiet'. Her father subsequently died following a heart attack and, due to the time associations, the child believed she had caused the death because she had failed to 'be quiet' when asked. It was perceived as her fault.

In another case, an eight-year-old boy was told by his mother to run next door and ask the neighbour to send for an ambulance as his father had collapsed. The child, who was taught not to go outside without changing into shoes, took off his slippers before running next door. On his return he was convinced he had caused the death of his father because he had been too slow.

Teachers make special provision for children whose first language is not English. This involves curriculum planning at school and English as an Additional Language (EAL) support. Teachers also work with the child's parents to determine whether they have special educational needs or other needs, perhaps as a result of the way in which they came to be in the UK, such as asylum seekers or refugees. This may include seeking advice from local refugee or ethnic communities; working with educational psychologists; social workers, child and adolescent mental health; specialist mental health and counselling services. Children who have been traumatised may respond to communication techniques which allow them to express themselves. This might include individual or small-group play to help newly arrived children settle in. Play can also be used to help children make sense of their experiences and explore issues such as fear and trust. Children can be encouraged to write about themselves, their home country and present circumstances, keep a diary or make a scrapbook or picture book about themselves. Younger children can use paints and crayons to draw about themselves, working with adults to write down captions to their drawings. These techniques can help them develop an understanding of complex events and feelings and can help the professionals involved understand how to tailor communication provision appropriately.[24]

School counsellor
Many schools now employ experts in child care and development from backgrounds

in nursing or social work who, in addition, have counselling skills and offer a supportive child's welfare role. These school counsellor positions are compulsory for boarding schools. Key features to this role include: open access; non-judgemental; non-disciplinary; safe and the ability to offer quality time. They have highly developed skills in communicating with difficult challenging children and young people and recognise the need to keep safe professional boundaries. Young people can self-refer as their services are advertised and access should be private, safe, confidential and in a discreet area of the school. Their communication techniques include gaining trust by using empowering methods, such as empathy, simple language and soft voice tones. They use play to help the young person to speak openly, as seen in the example below. Other therapeutic tools include sand trays and the use of 'heroes' and 'villains' from age-appropriate books and films.

Use of play to create a home environment

An 11-year-old boy, one of twins, had neonatal difficulties that affected his speech and educational development. The trigger from teachers was a concern that there was neglect to one twin and favour to another at home, and yet there was no real evidence. Finally, after a period of time the neglected twin was encouraged to see the school counsellor. Using doll's house furniture the child acted out with the figures what was happening to him at home. He acted out being placed in the cupboard. He shut the doors and hit the cupboard and swore at it ('I hate you . . . you are . . .', etc.), he continued while punching the cupboard. As a result of this session he was referred to social services and the family was offered appropriate help.

The social worker

Social workers work with children with special educational needs and vulnerable children who may have been affected by adverse experiences (*see* previous section and Table 5.1, p. 59). Many children fail to trust any adult figure because of past abuse or neglect. Therefore, social workers have developed skills to enable these children and young people to talk about situations they suppress because they are emotionally painful by using counselling and psychological approaches.[25,26] In these communications social workers are vigilant and sensitive to the hidden suppressed world of the child. Skills and techniques are perceived in social work as transferrable individual attributes. Social work skills focus on developing personal capacity in promoting skilled communication with children; this is termed a 'capacity-building approach'.[4] The emphasis is on self-awareness and reflective practice. The social worker must develop trust before any communication can take place. Their focus is that the child is capable and aims to ensure an anti-oppressive framework. To build this type of relationship through which communication can begin is time-consuming. Clinical encounters with children where time is limited need to adopt approaches which build rapport quickly. The ability to do this depends upon a professional's insight and self-awareness, together with an ability to reflect upon their demeanour, body posture, voice tone and facial gestures. For this age range use of non-directive play is essential,[27,28] combined with the ability to praise and draw out positives from children who have rarely been placed in a positive light. Social workers may use or direct children and young people to Triangle (www.triangle.org.uk), an independent organisation that has developed skills training for professionals and advocates for child-centred communication.

Social worker

TOP TIPS

Use of non-verbal modes, child-centred techniques and approaches using play and geneograms, 'life story work', 'wishes and feelings'. Children prefer communication based on activity and short utterances within informal play settings. See the following 'key skills':

- respect/trust
- listening
- empathy
- summarising
- explaining
- consulting
- negotiating
- consistency.

The SCIE states that child-led communication involves (p. 24):

- allowing children to have some control over both the process and the content of the communication
- taking time to prepare children for their participation
- providing explanations about the process that they can understand
- offering choices regarding the extent of participation, with room for some compromise and negotiation
- demonstrating a sense of fairness
- giving support and encouragement.[4]

ADOLESCENT (12–18 YRS) = IDENTITY VERSUS ROLE CONFUSION

Adolescence is a time of physical and emotional change, a time of uncertainty, especially about identity, all of which can become manifest in mood swings and challenging communication. WHO classifies young people as 10–24 years old and adolescence as 10–19 years of age.[29]

The school nurse

The school nurses' remit is expanding within preventative and public health. They spend time working with young people helping them to understand their bodily changes and develop mature insights into health and well-being.

School nurses
TOP TIPS

- Be open and honest.
- Circular open seating positions.
- Give space as adolescents usually do not like to be crowded.
- Understand their language and their use of colloquialisms (e.g. 'last night was really sick' meaning really, really good), but beware – usage changes constantly!
- Dress code matters and many professionals want to be able to wear jeans when working with adolescents.
- Make time – consultations must not be rushed.
- Be open about confidentiality and what is and must be shared with a teacher and what can be concealed.
- Set up boxes for posting questions as face-to-face communication may not be possible.
- Use IT, including email, websites, social networking sites and texting, etc.
- Advertise in an appropriate way, for example imaginative use of the Internet.

The nurse practitioner or practice nurse

Some young people have regular contacts with practice nurses who monitor long-term chronic health problems such as asthma. Young people frequently choose the nurse for disclosure of problems and worries, especially if they cannot see a GP of the same sex and are fearful about confidentiality.[30] Local programmes in which young people have been encouraged to consult with their practice nurse have led to significant findings with disclosures on health concerns, identification of risk behaviours and mental health problems. The need for confidentiality and consent training are key themes in the success of such projects.[31] In particular confidence to declare with clarity to the young person what will be written down and how (normally agreed with the young person and shown them) and who else will have access to this information.

The school counsellor

School counsellors work in high schools and private access for students is a key requirement of their role. The environment and approach especially with young people must promote a feeling of safety and privacy.

School counsellor's approach to working with young people

➤ Setting up the environment: this might include beanbags for floor seating, use of different art materials, calming objects such as shells and pebbles, use of neutral colours of nature and sea.
➤ The meeting: create a relaxed informal atmosphere using first name terms. Clear explanations on role and confidentiality (information will be shared if a young person is seen to be at risk and this must be clear from the outset).

Opening sentences, 'I am here to work with young people who have worries about school or home or both, I wonder if that's why you have come to see me – this is your time. I am here to listen and help'; 'Has the teacher sent you?' As conversation progresses care must be taken about references to the home environment. For example,

Counsellor: Who's living at home?
Adolescent: I have a brother
Counsellor: Oh, is he at school?

➤ Content: aim to engage the young person and gain their trust. This may be difficult with those who say very little. In these situations a magic box may be used (*see* Figures 5.1 and 5.2). Start the game by playing in any open space and ask them to play with you. The box can be a good ice-breaker for those children or young people who are silent. The counsellor will pick up neutral items and reflect on them. Each item selected will be about someone they know (e.g. the counsellor might pick up a bright object and say, 'This bright little marble makes me think of my youngest daughter who likes to wear bright pink clothes'), the object is then placed on the table. What they select and why can reveal a great deal of the child's background (e.g. an absent parent, a sick or ill sibling, an abusive grandparent, etc.).

➤ Conclusion: sessions end with open continued access negotiated and enabled. Often an item from the magic box can be given to the child to take away and bring back to establish the ongoing connection and access. Access might be given via email.

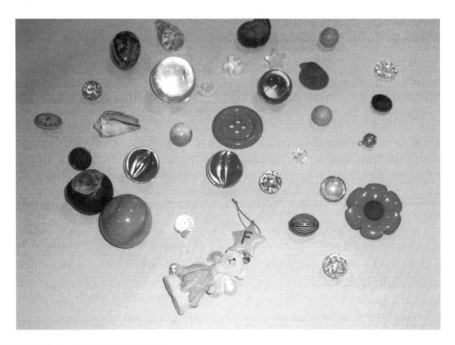

FIGURE 5.1 Magic box items

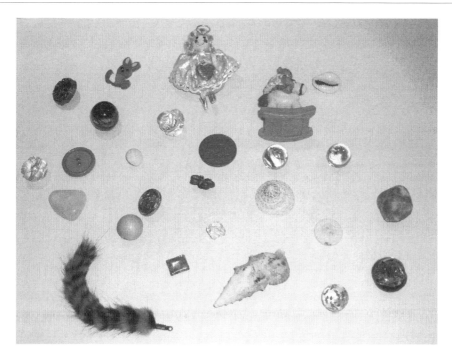

FIGURE 5.2 Magic box items

Case of young female aged 13 years

A young girl aged 13 years self-referred to a school counsellor because she was struggling with friendship groups and focusing in class. She describes how her teachers had not identified the problem although her grades had deteriorated. She was struggling with a chronic alcoholic father, a brother with bipolar disease and the young girl did not want to be an added burden on her mother, who was a teacher, trying to hold the family together. The young girl failed to share her worries with her mother. However, she could not sleep, was feeling anxious, having problems with her peer group, and feeling stressed and worried about school work and her poor grades. The counsellor helped her understand that her family situation was not her fault and also explained the dynamics of alcohol abuse and co-dependency. The counsellor provided refuge, security and opportunity to talk through her worries, to enable her to develop strategies to cope. The counsellor was also able to flag up support in the classroom without disclosing information given in confidence to the teachers.

The social worker

The social worker works with young people in a range of ways; for example, in community engagement projects; in the care of vulnerable and looked-after young people; those in foster and residential care, secure accommodation or in therapeutic communities; and with disabled young people. A great deal of literature on effective communication with this age group comes from looked-after children.[32] The social work approach to communication with this age range is framed with respect for what the young person can do, consideration of their needs and their rights, a focus on stepping into the young person's shoes, an acceptance for who they are and a concern to hear their views and consider their future.[33] In all these situations social work finds itself listening to the voice of young people and seeking to make partnership decisions with them. Success depends upon trust and commitment and young people have asked professionals working with them to:

➤ be on time and don't cancel unless you have to
➤ invest time in getting to know them
➤ be honest
➤ do what you say you will do (e.g. keep promises)
➤ show interest in the positives as well as the problems
➤ be responsive to what young people say
➤ believe in their capabilities.[33]

In gaining trust social workers draw upon transference and counter-transference, developing an environment where young people feel safe to communicate openly, often using techniques of mirroring, empathy and 'attunement'.[34] The ability to use objects which have meaning and hold the young person's interest, such as computer games or a family pet, can help build connections; also the use of poetry, reading, artwork and drama or valuable aids to unlock their thinking.

Listening to young people's voices and achieving inclusive participation has resulted in recent changes to practice, much of which has been propelled through the work of the voluntary sector, such as Save the Children and the Children's Society. These bodies have helped to frame guidance for effective partnership decision-making with young people.[35]

Skills required for decision-making with young people

- Share all the information so that young people are informed to make decisions.
- Give time and explanation for understanding.
- Have ongoing meetings if required (do not confine a decision to one meeting).
- Use an appropriate setting which is comfortable, private and culturally appropriate.
- Give the young person time to prepare beforehand and think things through afterwards to consider the 'What if?' questions.
- Focus on the young person's priorities.
- Give them access to an advocate or supporter.
- Pay attention to any special needs.
- Give feedback on discussions concerning the outcome of the decision as many young people feel listened to but often unable to influence the outcome.

INTERPROFESSIONAL WORKING AND INTERPROFESSIONAL COMMUNICATION RELATING TO CHILDREN AND YOUNG PEOPLE

Many of the different professionals discussed so far in this chapter work together to care for children and their families. Joint working enables the sharing of different skills and expertise often across professional boundaries, for example from health to education and social care. This collaborative working is underpinned by effective interprofessional communication.[36] On a day-to-day working level these communications result in the sharing of different profession-specific working practices. For example, the doctor may share physiological details of the deteriorating health of an infant with a health visitor, who relates back to the doctor insights from the home environment or emotional state of the mother. These perspectives in combination help to inform individual professional practice and form an agreed joint management plan for the child and family. In some instances the quality of the communication exchanged between different professionals can be inadequate to some degree. This may be for several reasons: the detail of the information exchanged is unclear and confusing, the communication is not face-to-face and there are missed non-verbal clues which prevent each party fully understanding the message, the communication is second-hand, and problems with acceptance due to poor working relationships and lack of trust. Although in essence straightforward, Whittington (2003) has argued that these interprofessional relationships need to be understood to ensure collaboration takes place. Effective interprofessional collaboration appears to require practitioners to learn, negotiate and apply understanding of what is common to the professions involved, their distinctive contributions and what is complementary between them, what may be in conflict, and how to work together (p. 58).[37]

Communicating interprofessionally on separate tasks relating to our different roles and responsibilities is an integrated activity that necessitates a level of shared understanding and mutual investment. This is much more clearly an interactive process than simply working in ways which are complementary and do not involve any significant degree of collaborative engagement. Earlier interprofessional team discussions regarding the confirmation of birth outcomes would have led to earlier support for the following example.

Example of interprofessional perspectives

The parents were concerned following a term emergency Caesarean section for their second child, a girl, due to fetal distress in labour. No concern was noted following birth by the obstetrician, paediatrician or midwife. Normal discharge from hospital led to the handover to the health visitor (HV) who recorded normal growth and development. However, at 16 months she had not started to walk (her brother walked at 18 months) but in addition, almost overnight, her speech stopped and her hands became weaker and started to begin flapping movements. Her HV sent her to the GP who sent her to a consultant paediatrician. She was found to have a small head and diagnosed with cerebral palsy due to oxygen starvation at birth. She was offered community physiotherapy. It took time for this service to be started. Immediately, the physiotherapist was not happy with the diagnosis and wrote to

> the paediatrician to see her again and asking for consideration of Rett's syndrome. She was referred back to the hospital consultant who sent her to the genetics department where Rett's syndrome was confirmed. The little girl then received more effective interprofessional case reviews and appropriate planned team working began.

Fully interprofessional working requires participants to be prepared in a number of ways. They must know about the roles of other professional groups, they must be able to work with other professionals in the context of a team, and they should be ready to substitute for roles traditionally played by other professionals when this would improve processes and outcomes for service.[38] Interprofessional education (IPE), where learners from different professional disciplines learn 'with, from and about each other to improve the quality of patient care', should embrace learning about effective team working and collaborative practice, as well as learning how to collaborate and work with others.[39] IPE in this way is perceived as a solution to help professionals learn to 'work together'.[40]

Meads and Ashcroft emphasise that 'learning about collaboration is one thing: learning how to collaborate is quite another. It is active-interaction between the parties who need to collaborate' that is required.[36] It is in interprofessional practice that relationships are developed and mutual trust developed. One example of interactive shared learning that has helped practitioners engage in difficult consultations with children and young people involves group sharing using Balint group techniques (from the work of Michael Balint, a psychoanalyst; p. 3).[35] In these groups a primary care team meet together and share their different experiences of communications with young people, reflecting and debating on how to progress each case. More interprofessional post-qualified courses are required on communication with children and young people.[41] The Bercow Report recommends that 'professionals across the children's and young people's workforce understand pre-qualification training in collaborative multidisciplinary working, alongside professionals from other backgrounds' (Recommendation 20, p. 9).[23]

Joint working assessment frameworks are emerging offering the potential for greater transparency concerning jointly held knowledge about the child and leading to fewer repeated communications with children and their families. The Common Assessment Framework (CAF) for children has yet to be fully embraced and its use varies nationally. The website has examples of where practitioners have used aspects of the framework.[42] One of the desired outcomes for the skills and knowledge for the Children's Workforce is to use CAF interprofessionally. It is a proactive tool for use in non-high-risk situations where there is no concern for harm or risk. It was designed to work in partnership with a designated lead professional, who acts as a single point of contact for the child and family and who works interprofessionally to enhance planned care.

CONCLUSION

This chapter has considered the skills used for communication by a range of different professionals working with children and young people, primarily in the community. The opportunity for progressing the skill base of those who work with children and young people through combining the range of expertise is enormous, especially if merged with the expertise of medicine (*see* Chapter 3, 4). Working together to realise the principles for effective communication, seen as 'common core' skills for the Children's Workforce, should ensure a child- and family-focused service, where the rights of children are identified and assessed using the skills of the individual professional and the pooled knowledge and skills of the collective Children's Workforce.[2,3,43] It is of concern, however, that children and young people are only just being asked to play a role in shaping policy. This is particularly important in health, as young people's perspectives differ from those of adults.[44] Hearing children's voices will depend upon them becoming more involved through the Patient Advice and Liaison Service (PALS), which in turn depends upon more effective communication channels with children and young people regarding their health and social care with all statutory and voluntary services.[45] This is indeed within the scope and vision of the new 2020 Children's and Young People's Workforce Strategy.[46]

Common themes

The insights of different professional groups provide common agreements on the skills required for communication with children:

➤ Focus only on the child or young person as the centre of the communication: every discipline works to hear the child's story, from being in tune with the baby, to playful activity with the toddler and young child, to eliciting dialogue with young people through using a range of techniques and approaches.

➤ Build empathy and trust: from the gentle handling of the baby, to the nursery nurse and health visitors getting in touch with the toddler's world, to the atmosphere created for young people by school counsellors, social workers and others.

➤ Understand the effects of non-verbal communication: from the facial expressions encouraged in mother–infant contact by the midwife, to the patience of the nursery nurse with toddlers, to the school nurse who uses IT and dresses in a professional but approachable way to make young people feel safe.

➤ Develop open honest relationships: from the social work approach of empowerment to the counsellors' ability to access powerful emotions and yet ensure permission to share conversations with relevant others.

➤ Be calm and non-threatening: from the soft tones to be used with baby, to the sensitive ability of the health visitor to judge when eye contact with the toddler can take place, to the motivation and belief of teachers in maximising every child's potential.

➤ Choose words with care: from communication with toddlers whose cognitions differ from those of adults, to the avoidance of professional acronyms, to selecting words and phrases which open up the black box as seen by the school counsellor and social worker who use play techniques and effective open questions.

➤ Listen: this is more than just comprehending what is said. All professions need to observe every mood change and behaviour pattern, which might speak louder than words.

➤ Use each other: interprofessional working can help as each professional shares different moments with children and young people and the collective wisdom is worth acquiring.

ACKNOWLEDGEMENTS

Health visitor and school nurse students, De Montfort University, 2008–9: Maureen Hill, Janet Graham, Ruth Gregg, Rachel Wandera, Lynn Wilkinson, Maria Turner, Sarah Fenwick, Chrisoula Jones, Jill Gullidge, Elaine Worden, Belinda Wright, Deborah Daw, Helen Symons, Donna Southwell.

Rose Griffiths, senior lecturer and National Teaching Fellow, School of Education University of Leicester.

Pen Green Centre for Children and Young Families (Research, Development and Training Base and Leadership Centre, Corby Northamptonshire www.pengreen. org/pengreencenter.php), particularly Dr Margy Whalley (director of Research and Development) and Tracy Gallagher (deputy head, Years 0–3).

Jane Gamble, school counsellor, Leicestershire.

Ali Tempest, speech and language therapist, senior lecturer, Faculty Health and Life Sciences, De Montfort University.

REFERENCES

1 Erikson EH. Childhood and society. In: Gross R. *Psychology the Science of Mind and Behaviour*. 2nd ed. East Kilbride: Hodder & Stoughton; 1992: 624–6.

2 Department for Education and Skills (DfES). *Common Core of Skills and Knowledge for the Children's Workforce*. Nottingham: DfES; 2005.

3 Department for Education and Skills (DfES). *Every Child Matters*. London: The Stationery Office; 2003.

4 Social Care Institute for Excellence (SCIE). *Social Work Education Knowledge Review 12: teaching, learning and assessing communication skills with children and young people in social work education*. London: SCIE; 2006.

5 Hodges V, Morgan L, Johnston B. Educating for excellence in child welfare practice: a model for graduate training in intensive family preservation. *J Teach Soc Work*. 1993; 7(1): 31–48.

6 Trowell J. The importance of observational training: an evaluative study. *International Journal of Infant Observation and its Applications*. 1998; 2(1): 101–11.

7 Lefevre M, Tanner K, Luckock B. Developing social work students' communication skills

with children and young people: a model for the qualifying level curriculum. *Child Fam Soc Work.* 2007; **13**: 166–76.

8 Nursing and Midwifery Council (NMC). *Standards of Proficiency for Specialist Community Public Health Nurses.* London: NMC; 2004.

9 Kent G, Dalgleish M. Early social relationships. In: Kent G, Dalgleish M. *Psychology and Medical Care.* London: WB Saunders; 1996. Chapter 6.

10 Businessballs. *Conscious Competence Learning Model.* Available at: www.businessballs.com/consciouscompetencelearningmodel.htm (access 15 June 2010).

11 Brazelton TB, Tronick E, Adamson K, *et al.* Early mother–infant reciprocity (1975). In: Kent G, Dalgleish M. *Psychology and Medical Care.* London: WB Saunders; 1996. Chapter 6.

12 Bowlby J. *Attachment and Loss: attachment.* Harmondsworth, Middlesex: Penguin Books; 1975. p. 1.

13 Rutter M. Clinical implications of attachment concepts: retrospect and prospect. *J Child Psychol Psyc.* 1995; **36**(4): 549–71.

14 Bowlby J. *A Secure Base: parent–child attachment and healthy human development.* Tavistock Professional Book. London: Routledge; 1988.

15 Ainsworth M, *et al. Deprivation of Maternal Care: a reassessment of its effects.* Geneva: World Health Organization, Public Health Papers, No. 14; 1962.

16 Bailey B. Parent–child relationships: developing a brief attachment-screening tool. *Community Pract.* 2009; **82**(3): 22–6.

17 Murray L, Andrews L. *The Social Baby: understanding babies' communication from birth.* Richmond: CP Publishing; 2007.

18 Cole M. Culture in development. In: Faulkner D, Littleton K, Woodhead M (editors). *Cultural Worlds of Early Childhood.* London: Routledge; 2004. Chapter 6.

19 Dorman H, Dorman C. Richmond: the children's project. In: Dorman H, Dorman C. *The Social Toddler: promoting positive behaviour.* Richmond: CP Publishing; 2004.

20 Webb N. Play and expressive therapies to help bereaved children: individual, family and group treatments. *Smith Coll Stud.* 2003; **73**(3): 405–22.

21 Griffiths R. Coping with bereavement In: Moyles J (editor). *Early Years Foundations: meeting the challenge.* Maidenhead: Open University Press; 2007. Chapter 7, pp. 105–20.

22 Royal College of Speech and Language Therapists. *I CAN – helps children communicate.* Available at: www.ican.org.uk/frontpage.aspx (accessed 15 June 2010).

23 Department for Children, Schools and Families (DCSF). *The Bercow Report: a review of services for children and young people (0–19) with speech, language and communication needs.* Nottingham: DCSF; 2008. Available at: www.dcsf.gov.uk/bercowreview/docs/7771-DCSF-BERCOW.PDF (accessed 15 June 2010).

24 Department of Education and Skills (DfES). *Aiming High: guidance on supporting the education of asylum seeking and refugee children.* Nottingham: DfES; 2004. Available at: www.standards.dfes.gov.uk/ethnicminorities/links_and_publications/AH_Gdnc_AS_RFG_Apr04/asylumguidance.pdf (accessed 15 June 2010).

25 Bell M. Promoting children's rights through the use of relationship. *Child Fam Soc Work.* 2002; **7**(1): 1–11.

26 De Winter M, Noom M. Someone who treats you as a normal human being . . .: homeless youth examine the quality of professional care. *Brit J Soc Work.* 2003; **33**(3): 325–38.

27 Thomas N, O'Kane C. Discovering what children think: connections between research and practice. *Brit J Soc Work.* 2000; **30**(6): 819–35.

28 McLeod A. *Listening but Not Hearing: barriers to effective communication between young people in public care and their social workers.* Lancaster: University of Lancaster; 2000.

29 Viner R, Booy R. Epidemiology of health and illness. *Brit Med J.* 2005: **19**(330); 411–14. Available at: www.ncbi.nlm.nih.gov/pmc/articles/PMC549118/ (accessed 30 June 2010).

30 Donovan C, Suckling H. *Difficult Consultations with Adolescents.* Oxford: Radcliffe Medical Press; 2004. p. 67.

31 Bell J. Case A: 'Anne' – the adolescent who will not speak. In: Donovan C, Suckling H, *et al. Difficult Consultations with Adolescents.* Oxford: Radcliffe Medical Press; 2004. Chapter 2, p. 78.

32 Krueger M, Stuart C. Context and competence in work with children and youth. *Child Youth Care Forum.* 1999; **28**(3): 195–204.

33 National Children's Bureau, Voice for the Child in Care (VCC). *Start with the Child, Stay with the Child: a blueprint for a child-centred approach to children and young people in public care.* London: VCC; 2005. p. 49. Available at: www.voiceyp.org/docimages/28.pdf (accessed 15 June 2010).

34 Ringel S. Play and impersonation: finding the right intersubjective rhythm. *Clin Soc Work J.* 2003; **31**(4): 371–81.

35 McNeish D, Newman T, Roberts H. *What Works for Children?* Buckingham: Open University Press; 2002. p. 196.

36 Meads G, Ashcroft J. *The Case for Interprofessional Collaboration.* Oxford: CAIPE Blackwell Publishing; 2005. Chapter 2, p. 15.

37 Whittington C. A model of collaboration. In: Weinstein J, Whittington C, Leiba T (editors). *Collaboration in Social Work Practice.* London: Jessica Kingsley Publishers; 2003; Chapter 2, pp. 39–62.

38 Hammick M, Freeth D, Copperman J, *et al. Being Interprofessional.* Cambridge: Polity Press; 2009. p. 9.

39 Freeth D, Hammick M, Reeves S, *et al. Effective Interprofessional Education, Development, Delivery and Evaluation.* Oxford: Blackwell, CAIPE; 2005.

40 World Health Organization. *Learning Together to Work Together for Health.* Technical Report Series No. 534. Geneva: World Health Organization; 1987.

41 Priest H, Sawyer A, Roberts P, *et al.* A survey of interprofessional education in communication skills in healthcare programmes in the UK. *J Interprof Care.* 2005; **19**(3): 236–50.

42 Department for Children Schools and Families (DfES). *The Common Assessment Framework for Children and Young People.* London: DfES; 2006. Available at: www.dcsf.gov.uk/every childmatters/strategy/deliveringservices1/caf/cafframework/ (accessed 15 June 2010).

43 Department of Health. *The National Service Framework for Children, Young People and Maternity Services.* London: DoH; 2004.

44 Liabo K, Curtis K, Toberts H, *et al. Health Futures: a consultation with children and young people in Camden and Islington about their experiences of receiving health services.* London: Camden and Islington Health Authority; 2002.

45 Roberts H. Children's participation in policy matters. In: Hallett C, Prout A. *Hearing the Voices of Children: social policy for the new century.* Oxon: RoutledgeFalmer; 2003.

46 Department for Children, Schools and Families (DCSF). *2020 Children and Young People's Workforce Strategy.* Nottingham: DCSF; 2008.

CHAPTER 6

Listening to young carers and their families

Jo Aldridge

INTRODUCTION

> People tend to protect children and young people. For me this translated into
> ignoring my need to be informed and involved. I needed someone to talk to
> who would listen in confidence and help me to express and explore the com-
> plex feelings and situations I was dealing with.[1]

The needs of young carers* in a healthcare consultation are as modest and uncompli-
cated as Marlowe describes above. Research studies to date have identified consistent
patterns in the nature and extent of young carers' needs, specifically the need for
these children and young people to have access to professionals who will listen to
them without making value judgements about their lives or threatening family status
and continuity.[2–4] However, ensuring young carers are consulted at all, never mind
in ways that address their needs as children and as carers, has presented a number
of challenges in both health and social care contexts. The complexity of meeting
these dual needs often results in gaps in service provision. Outside school, general
practice is often the first point at which young carers could present or be identified
as children with distinct health and/or social care needs. Furthermore, GPs are ideally placed to implement preventive strategies for patients and their families. For
example, in their study of the role of primary care in the management of adolescent
mental health problems, Kramer and Garralda (2000) found that the trust families
place in GPs means that they are ideally placed to implement feasible and effective
interventions.[5]

---

* Young carers are children under the age of 18 who care for a sick or disabled relative (usually a parent) in the home (*see* Becker S. Young carers. In: Davies M (editor). *The Blackwell Encyclopaedia of Social
Work*. Oxford: Blackwell; 2000; p. 378).

There are estimated to be around 175 000 children and young people in the UK who are providing care for a sick or disabled relative at home.[6] Many of these children are caring for parents who have physical or mental health problems which can be combined with substance misuse problems. While young carers are clearly a small sub-group of vulnerable children in the UK, current estimates of the numbers are understated because many families affected by parental disability or illness do not disclose the fact that their children are having to provide care.[4] Furthermore, it has been argued that a critical factor in the identification of children as carers is the onset of parental disability or chronic illness.[7,8] Thus, estimates about the numbers of young carers nationally should take account of statistics on parental disability – current evidence suggests that three million children in the UK live in families where chronic illness or disability is present.[9]

The main focus of empirical investigation and policy and practice interventions to date has been on the impact of caring on children and their families. In many respects, this is a critical aspect in understanding and supporting children as carers. A young carer's perspective – which has taken as its focus a children's rights approach – does not then suggest all children of parents with illness or disability are carers, but that parental impairment can be a potential trigger for the onset of young caring. This approach also recognises that when caring by children becomes long term, or disproportionate to their age and level of maturity, it can compromise their successful transitions into adulthood.[10] Research has shown consistently that when caring becomes long term, incommensurate with age and ability and is unsupported, this has a detrimental impact on children's lives in respect of their educational attainment, their emotional health and well-being and their transitions into adulthood.[3,4,11–13]

The type of responsibilities that children undertake can be wide-ranging. For example, many children undertake domestic responsibilities such as household management, cooking and cleaning as well as nursing duties such as administering medication and toileting parents. These aspects of young carers' lives have only been revealed through empirical investigations that have involved talking directly with children and young people about their responsibilities and experiences when parents have an illness or disability.[14] Prior to the early young carers' studies in the 1990s, many children continued to care unsupported because practitioners rarely talked to them about their experiences, even though their parents were often in receipt of support services from a range of health and social care providers.[2,15] Consider this account of one young carer from one of the earliest pieces of research in this field:

> When I think about all those years I cared for my dad, it makes me angry, not because I had to care for him – I wanted to care for him – but because I was left alone to cope with his illness for so long. I wasn't just doing ordinary tasks like other kids might do around the house. I was having to cook for him, beg for money and food parcels so I could feed him, take him to the toilet. All I ever wanted was to talk to someone and someone who could have warned me about my dad's fits, caused by his brain tumour.[2]

In respect of further studies that have looked at the needs of these children, and particularly the implications for health and social care practitioners, it is clear that age-appropriate and sensitive interventions are required that focus on consulting with these children in ways that are child-centred and non-threatening.[3,4] One of the first studies of children who care for parents with serious mental health problems used qualitative methodology to explore the views of 40 young carers, their parents and a range of professionals involved in providing services to these families.[7] The authors suggest that '[p]rofessionals need to reconcile children's fear of professional interventions with their need for formal support. Children need to talk to someone they can trust and who understands their needs – as children and as carers'.[7]

YOUNG CARERS: DUALITY AND TENSIONS

Research studies on young carers have identified the need to have someone to talk to as a critical and consistent finding. This has obvious and direct implications for the consultation process in healthcare settings with vulnerable children; but it also presents some key challenges for practitioners. One of these challenges is the duality or conflict inherent in the young caring experience, which is manifest in a number of ways. First, the polarity between children's status and experience when they care is represented in interventions that aim to safeguard and protect children from harm on the one hand and approaches to young caring on the other that result in practitioners either overlooking or condoning children's responsibilities as carers. Consequently, young carers have tended to fall between the gaps in service provision for children and (adult-centred) interventions aimed at carers.

Second, young carers may present to primary or secondary healthcare services simply as the children of patients, when in fact they are often the carers of parents (patients) who are ill or disabled. Research on triadic communication in primary care paediatric consultation has shown that children aged 6–12 years are usually accompanied by an adult carer during consultation with GPs.[16] In respect of young carers, the situation is often reversed, although practitioners may not be aware of children's change in roles in their consultations with adult patients. Young carers often accompany their parents when visiting GPs or hospitals for a number of reasons; these may include the need for children to assist parents with their physical impairments, or helping parents who have language difficulties. Young carers are often overlooked as potential patients or service users themselves in these contexts.[12,17] On the other hand, children may themselves present with symptoms that occur as a direct consequence of caring. For example, physical injuries associated with lifting a disabled parent or emotional difficulties are not uncommon among young carers.[18] However, they may not disclose their caring role to GPs and will not do so without appropriate and sensitive interventions that do not threaten personal or family stability.

Research on children who care for parents with mental health problems has shown that voluntary workers or community social or mental health workers are more likely to be identified as key professionals in their lives than GPs.[7] Even GPs who are well known to their patients and visit the family home to administer treatment tend to overlook the needs of children even when it is clear that no other parent or adult carer is living in the family home. Consider the following from a young carer who looked after her sister as well as her bedridden mother: '[the GP] only really stopped five minutes. She just come and had a look, told me mum that she'd got to start coming off antibiotics a bit and just went again'.[7]

Young caring also presents challenges and tensions in respect of current thinking about the sociology of childhood, which sees children as active and competent social agents.[19] In many respects, young carers demonstrate their competency and adaptability daily with the type of responsibilities they undertake and which we usually associate with adulthood. However, such proficiency is often precocious or incongruent with other childhood experiences or abilities and may, if allowed to continue unsupported, have long-term implications for children's emotional health and well-being. This may in turn compromise their potential for engaging in the kind of active citizenship in which their peers may participate. Furthermore, the participation agenda is key in respect of social welfare approaches to childhood and is based on international legislation that promotes participation as a fundamental principle of children's human rights.

A number of policy documents have recommended that children should be encouraged by health practitioners to express their views (as patients) and to participate in decisions made about care plans and services.[20,21] The National Service Framework (NSF) (2004) for children places children at the centre of their care as patients in primary care consultations. The recommendations in the NSF include promoting children's active involvement in decisions about their own health and the provision of appropriate information and reminders about consent procedures.[22] However, there is no reason why this should not also extend to children who are carers, who may need help and support either as patients, as carers or both. In fact, to ensure the needs of young carers are met effectively and appropriately, it is essential that practitioners adopt rights-based and holistic, whole family, approaches to consultation processes. In the case of children who care, this would mean that GPs, for example, should offer individual consultations with children as well as triadic interventions, as appropriate.[23] This would mean that where GPs suspect children may be taking on caring responsibilities for ill or disabled adults, or when children or parents themselves have disclosed this information, then dedicated support should be offered to these children, including one-to-one consultations if this is deemed appropriate by parents and children themselves.

In many respects, young caring can present a number of challenges to a rights-based, participative approach. For example, on the one hand, as Göpfert and colleagues (1996) argue, 'it is the right of children to deal with [worries about his/her parents] by caring for their parent';[24] on the other hand, many children do not want to care to the extent that they do, if at all, and as children they should have the right to stop caring if that is what they wish. This is especially important when caring has a detrimental impact on children's health, well-being and development, something that will be of crucial concern to the primary healthcare practitioner. Research has shown us that many children do not want to undertake the kinds of intimate caring tasks, such as bathing and toileting their parents, that they and their parents often find so embarrassing.[15] However, it is only by talking to children and their families about their needs in this respect that interventions will help address their rights and needs as children and as carers effectively.

This has been a fundamental message from the numerous qualitative studies that have put children's views and voices at the forefront of methodological approaches in social care research. These conclusions help inform, if not transform, consultative processes in healthcare settings (a point which will be discussed in more detail later). In such contexts, it is only by understanding and addressing young carers' needs both as carers and as children – as children in need and/or as patients – that advances will be made in consultative processes between practitioners and this group of vulnerable children. As Hill and colleagues (2004) have argued, only if 'genuine dialogue occurs between children and the adults in power' will policies and services 'respond to children's felt needs, rather than to needs attributed to them'.[25]

RECOGNITION, IDENTIFICATION AND TRAINING

A number of studies on children's participation in primary healthcare consultations point to a growing need for improved multi-agency work.[5] This is also true in respect of healthcare interventions for young carers and these should include better measures for recognising and identifying young carers and for healthcare practitioners, particularly in primary healthcare services, to make appropriate referrals and work alongside other agencies that may be able to offer dedicated services to these children.[24,25] Identifying the specific consultation skills and training requirements health practitioners need in order to work effectively with young carers is vital but to date has acquired little attention. In many respects, social care interventions (and policies) have identified and addressed the needs of young carers and their families in the UK,[26] but success in this field has not necessarily extended to healthcare settings, particularly in primary healthcare services.

Currently, in the UK, young carers can be assessed as children in need under the Children Act 1989 or as carers, alongside their ill or disabled parents, under the Carers (Recognition and Services) Act 1995; and with reference to the principles set out in the Framework for Assessment of Children in Need and their Families. Many voluntary agency practitioners and particularly Young Carers Project workers also undertake needs assessments using their own assessment tools and measures.[27] However, while social care interventions through social services and voluntary organisations such as young carers' projects and children's charities have developed tools to work more effectively with young carers, identification of children's caring roles and recognition of their needs in healthcare settings continue to be problematic.

Research suggests that primary healthcare practitioners, particularly GPs, often overlook the needs of young carers.[7,28] There are a number of possible reasons for such oversights. First, the responsibility for such omissions does not always lie with health practitioners themselves. The reluctance among children and parents to disclose the fact that children are providing care for parents in the home is well documented.[11,12] Research has shown consistently that children are wary of presenting to health and social services as carers because they fear safeguarding and child protection decisions will be made that could lead to family separations.[4,9]

The reasons why young carers' needs are overlooked by health professionals may also lie in lack of time and resources to focus on children's needs as carers rather than the needs of adult patients. Research in other areas of primary healthcare practice has also recognised these constraints. For example, in their study of childhood obesity and primary care interventions, Walker and colleagues (2007), found that, 'time constraint, lack of training and lack of resources' were identified by GPs and practice nurses as significant factors in their ability to consult with children effectively on obesity issues.[29] Research on young caring has shown consistently that GPs and health practitioners in adult services do not see consultation with their patients' children as part of their professional responsibility, even when confronted in the home with adult patients being cared for in the main by their children.[7] Furthermore, evidence has also shown that GPs are often uncertain about how best to respond to young carers because of the lack of appropriate training opportunities and dedicated young carers' services to which to refer these children.[2,7]

Where parents suffer from mental health problems evidence also suggests that health and social care practitioners make assumptions about the risks to children, without discussing these with the family. Many also make assumptions about children's cognitive abilities or level of understanding about health issues and particular conditions.[7] It was clear from the young carers and parental mental illness study that practitioners, including GPs and mental health professionals, often assumed children were at risk of significant harm or developmental delay when parents had serious mental health problems. These assumptions were made without talking to children themselves and the presumed consequences for children of living with a parent with mental illness were wholly negative and detrimental to children's experiences and development. The authors concluded, 'professional understanding about the effects of parental mental illness on children are, in the main, based on assumptions – as well as the messages from child protection and joint working within a legal framework – rather than on any direct evidence through close contact with families'.[7]

In their review of research on primary care paediatric consultation, described in an earlier chapter, Cahill and Papageorgiou (2007) found that children had little measurable involvement in consultations and 'are unlikely to participate in the treatment planning and discussion parts of the consultation'.[23] The authors point to a convincing evidence base that suggests, 'children over the age of five years should be presumed competent to be involved in their own healthcare choices'. Once again, evidence of young caring often presents a challenge to, and conflicts with, practitioners' perceptions about children's ability and knowledge. In many respects, when children care the nature and extent of their responsibilities and the degree of close personal contact with parents and their health conditions means they often gain precipitate competencies, but because these are often learnt precociously and even unwittingly, while they can become skill rich, they often remain information poor.[2] Thus, on a day-to-day basis, children can learn to deal with their parents' illnesses or disabilities in accordance with the particular nature of the medical condition or impairment concerned and thus can even learn to anticipate their parents' health needs, but they often remain outside the sphere of intervention and care planning in respect of treatment and consultation with health practitioners.

Arguably, one of the main reasons for this oversight is lack of training and advice for practitioners. While guidance is available for professionals, including health practitioners, about how best to work with young carers and their families,[30] such guidance is often generalised and broadly based and has little grounding in evidence that provides insight into current GP consulting practices with young carers and their families. We also know little about the training and information needs of primary care practitioners in this respect. However, more recent strategies for improving the lives of young carers attempt to address this oversight. The National Carers' Strategy (2008) contains recommendations aimed at future support for young carers, including materials for GPs and hospital discharge teams to build awareness and skills in dealing with young carers.[31]

Primary healthcare services, particularly general practice, are often the first locations in which young carers come to the attention of healthcare practitioners. It is therefore essential that these professionals are able to recognise the triggers for young caring; to identify young carers in families where parents have chronic illness or disability; and to use appropriate tools, such as needs assessment protocols, to consult with them effectively. In many respects, the first two requisites point clearly to the need for awareness-raising strategies and training programmes for healthcare practitioners. This is congruent with government proposals that pledge support for young carers in respect of improving 'awareness training about young carers for GPs, primary healthcare teams [and subsequently] through providing opportunities for young carers to share their experiences with practitioners'.[30] At present it is not clear how these proposals will be formulated and implemented.

CONSULTING WITH YOUNG CARERS: MESSAGES FROM RESEARCH AND PRACTICE

In terms of consulting with young carers more effectively in healthcare settings, lessons can be learnt from new and innovative methodological approaches with vulnerable respondents in social science research, for example, as well as from consulting strategies that have proved effective in other areas of primary healthcare practice.

In many ways, research methodologies that adopt participative approaches with children can teach us a lot about how to work with children, and particularly vulnerable children, more effectively. Young carers do not always disclose details about their caring activity and their own health needs, during consultations. Sometimes they do not want to talk or feel too afraid to talk openly in contexts that are time restricted (such as the GP surgery) or because they fear professional interventions that may compromise family stability and continuity. This has also been the case in research with people who have learning disabilities, who often don't have the cognitive or verbal skills to participate in interviews or consultative, conversation-based dialogue. While researching these groups can often make the researcher break the 'rules' of ethnographic research,[32] they also present useful opportunities for developing new methods of elicitation to enable vulnerable respondents to 'open up'. Visual tools and prompts such as photographs and artwork are particularly useful in these contexts in that they provide respondents with the chance to show, rather than tell, their stories and experiences.[32,33] They are also congruent with the set of competences described in the Consultation Assessment and Improvement Instrument for Nurses (CAIIN), in particular consultation techniques that 'allow the patient to tell the story of their illness in their own words'.[34] Radley and Taylor (2003) used photographs taken by postoperative hospital patients to better understand the impacts of the hospital environment on patients' mood and recovery capacity.[35] They found that using photographs in this way provided 'a direct entry into [the respondent's] point of view . . . the technique of photography is a culturally fashioned extension of the senses . . . so that it provides a potential to question, arouse curiosity, tell in different voices, or see through different eyes from beyond'.[35]

These approaches have been mirrored also in a number of social care interventions for young carers. For example, a number of young carers' projects have developed assessment tools and progress-monitoring strategies based on visual rather than verbal techniques. Allowing children to take photographs in order to demonstrate visually their caring experiences have proved useful in these and other therapeutic contexts in that they allow children to develop their technical and artistic skills. This is not to suggest that such an approach would necessarily be appropriate or viable in terms of consultations with GPs. While time spent consulting with patients has increased among GP services in recent years, the 11.7-minute average time available to patients now still allows little time for GPs to address the often complex needs of young carers and their families.[36] While research on young caring has shown that sometimes all young carers need from either health or social care practitioners is 'a five minute phone call'[7] – often just to check that everything at home is all right or to make an appropriate referral – new and innovative methods of primary care paediatric consultation should also be considered.

Introducing such methods, including participative visual techniques, as part of a developing training package for primary care practitioners could help improve current consultation processes with young carers and their families and ensure that primary care services provide more effective early interventions in these families' lives. Providing information about referral procedures in respect of other health or social care agencies would be a key theme in any training programme aimed at primary care practitioners as well as an integral part of the consultation process itself, where young carers express a need for this and where these agencies are in place locally to provide this type of support.

Advances have been made in other areas of health and social care practice that have important implications and messages in the primary care context. In their review of interventions relating to child and adolescent mental health problems in primary care, Kramer and Garralda (2000) noted the success of family therapy clinics based in general practices,[5] an approach that finds resonance with the introduction in social care services of family group conferences for vulnerable children and families, including young carers. However, the authors warn of the high costs of setting up family clinics within GP services and the involvement of multidisciplinary teams of professionals, including psychiatrists and social workers. Nevertheless, the authors argue that primary care practitioners have an important role to play in adopting more holistic approaches, where 'combining attention to physical and emotional aspects is particularly appropriate'. Such an approach is particularly apposite in respect of addressing the needs of young carers and their families in primary care settings.

It is acknowledged that professionals working in these areas need access to new and targeted consulting skills training.[23] Where dedicated training has been offered to GPs, for example, evidence reveals improved consulting skills in a number of areas. Bernard and colleagues (1999) found that trainee GPs 'demonstrated improved self-perceived competence, knowledge and recognition of disorder' when offered single-session training on child and adolescent mental health.[37] Such a training package included preparatory reading and a teaching session that comprised problem-solving exercises, role play and the use of video vignettes. In respect of work with young carers, a number of agencies, including young carers' projects, have produced their own video resources to help raise awareness among health and social care practitioners about the experiences and needs of young carers and their families.[38]

A number of approaches are required in relation to consulting with young carers in primary care settings. In summary, a holistic (whole family) framework needs to include the following consultative principles and approaches.

Recognition and identification

GPs and other primary care practitioners need the skills to be able to recognise the triggers for young caring and to be able to identify children who may be undertaking primary care responsibilities in the home. Training programmes should include: information about trigger factors for the onset of care among children, safeguarding factors, understanding the impacts of caring on children and families, children's coping mechanisms and resilience factors. Information about these and other issues will help practitioners identify early young carers in primary healthcare settings.

Consultation in practice

Triadic and/or individual consultations with parents or children are required and non-threatening approaches that allow children (and parents) to talk openly and in confidence about their experiences and needs. In terms of understanding and listening, practitioners should consider adult patients' parenting experiences and needs. Young carers also require information about health conditions, diagnoses, prognoses and treatments. Participation is essential and practitioners should ensure that young carers are included in discussions about care plans, treatments and prognoses as well as their own needs. A number of assessment strategies and tools are used in social care to ensure that the needs of young carers and their families are met effectively. Training programmes should include information about how to use visual tools and prompts and other participatory approaches when consulting with young carers that enable them to talk more openly about their caring experiences. A number of video and DVD resources on young caring are also available for training purposes and many have been produced by young carers themselves. Information is also widely available about the type of practical support and assistance available to young carers as well as child-centred information about a wide range of medical health conditions and disabilities. Guidance on policy and needs assessments relating specifically to young carers is also available and should be an integral part of any training package on young caring.

Referral and multi-agency communication

Practitioners should also make appropriate referrals where necessary (and through discussion with young carers and families) to relevant agencies who may be able to offer dedicated support and help for young carers and their families as well as advice about benefits, practical aids and equipment, etc. There are more than 140 young carers' projects in the UK, many of which offer one-to-one support for young carers, as well as homework clubs, leisure activities and respite and befriending opportunities, etc. Making contact and working with professionals in other areas such as education and social services would also be useful in ensuring young carers have access to the range of support and help that they need. Training programmes should include information resources and links to young carers' projects in the UK, as well as details about the numbers and types of agencies and organisations that promote and support work with young carers and their families.

CONCLUSION

Research on young caring has shown that the needs of children when they care are often modest and need not be costly in terms of health and social care resources. Often children want someone they can talk to about their experiences and who will be reliable.[7] Kramer and Garralda (2000) argue that GPs are trusted by families, 'and are therefore in a position to provide them with information, support and advice. They may thus also be in a good position to implement preventive interventions'.[5] Preventing young caring is problematic for a number of reasons, not least because when there is no one else available to care, children undertake caring responsibilities through the fact of their availability as they share a home and because they want to help in some way and feel their contributions count. Parent–child bonds and attachment can also be enhanced through caring. In many respects, the role of GPs in supporting young carers is compromised by systemic constraints and lack of resources in other areas of health and social care provision. When parents are chronically ill or disabled, and particularly when they are parenting alone, they often have little choice but to call on the services of their child or children to care, because of the lack of alternative support services available. This is especially the case when parents need help and assistance at difficult times, for example during the night or in times of sudden crisis.

Currently, it is unclear how government strategies will address the specific needs of young carers and their families in terms of primary care service interventions. However, undoubtedly the role GPs and other health service practitioner's play in supporting young carers can be enhanced through the implementation of appropriate training strategies and improved consulting skills. Furthermore, generating debate and dialogue about new and innovative consulting practices in primary care is a fundamental first step in ensuring the needs of young carers and their families are fully recognised and met.

REFERENCES

1 Marlowe J. Helpers, helplessness and self-help. 'Shaping the silence': a personal account. In: Gopfert M, Webster J, Seeman MV (editors). *Parental Psychiatric Disorder: distressed parents and their families.* Cambridge: Cambridge University Press; 1996. pp. 135–51.

2 Aldridge J, Becker S. *Children Who Care: inside the world of young carers.* Loughborough: Young Carers Research Group; 1993.

3 Becker S, Aldridge J, Dearden C. *Young Carers and Their Families.* Oxford: Blackwell Science; 1998.

4 Meredith H. Young carers: the unacceptable face of community care. *Soc Work Soc Sci Rev.* 1991; Suppl. 3: 47–51.

5 Kramer T, Garralda ME. Child and adolescent mental health problems in primary care. *Adv Psychiatr Treat.* 2000; **6**: 287–94.

6 Office for National Statistics. *The Census in England and Wales.* Newport, South Wales: Office for National Statistics; 2001. Available at: www.statistics.gov.uk/Census2001/ (accessed 25 June 2010).

7 Aldridge J, Becker S. Children who care for parents with mental illness. In: Aldridge J, Becker S. *Perspectives of Young Carers, Parents and Professionals.* Bristol: The Policy Press; 2003.

8 Aldridge J, Wates M. Young carers and their disabled parents: moving the debate on. In: Newman T, Wates M (editors). *Disabled Parents and their Children: building a better future.* Ilford: Barnardos; 2004. pp. 80–95.

9 Dearden C, Aldridge J. Young carers: needs, rights and assessment. In: Horwath J (editor). *The Child's World: assessing children in need.* 2nd ed. London: Jessica Kingsley; 2009. pp. 214–28.

10 Dearden C, Becker S. *Growing up Caring: vulnerability and transitions to adulthood – young carers' experiences.* Leicester: Leicester Youth Work Press; 2000.

11 Dearden C, Becker S. *Young Carers in the United Kingdom: a profile.* London: Carers National Association; 1998.

12 Dearden C, Becker S. *Young Carers in the UK: the 2004 report.* London: Carers UK; 2004.

13 Frank J, Tatum C, Tucker S. *On Small Shoulders: learning from the experiences of former young carers.* London: Children's Society; 1999.

14 Bilsborrow S. *'You Grow Up Fast As Well . . .' Young carers on Merseyside.* Liverpool: Carers National Association, Personal Services Society, Barnardos; 1992.

15 Aldridge J, Becker S. *My Child, My Carer: the parents' perspective.* Loughborough: Young Carers Research Group; 1994.

16 Tates K, Elbers E, Meeuwesen L, Bensing J. Doctor–parent–child relationship: a 'pas de trois'. *Patient Educ Couns*. 2002, **48**: 5–14.

17 The Children's Society. *The National Young Carers Initiative*. 2009. Available at: www.young carer.com/showPage.php?file=index.htm (accessed 15 June 2010).

18 Hill S. The physical effects of caring on children. *Journal of Young Carers Work*. 1999; **3**: 6–7.

19 Wyness MG. *Childhood and Society: an introduction to the sociology of childhood*. Basingstoke: Palgrave MacMillan; 2006.

20 British Medical Association. *Consent, Rights and Choices in Health Care for Children and Young People*. London: British Medical Journal Books; 2000.

21 Alderson P, Montgomery J. *Health Care Choices: making decisions with children*. London: Institute for Public Policy Research; 1996.

22 Department of Health (DH). *Long Term Health Conditions 2009: research study conducted for the Department of Health*. London: DH; 2009. Available at: www.dh.gov.uk/en/Publicationsandstatistics/Publications/PublicationsPolicyAndGuidance/DH_101090 (accessed 15 June 2010).

23 Cahill P, Papageorgiou A. Triadic communication in the primary care paediatric consultation: a review of the literature. *Brit J Gen Pract*. 2007; **57**(544): 904–11.

24 Göpfert M, Webster J, Seeman MV (editors). *Parental Psychiatric Disorder: distressed parents and their families*. Cambridge: Cambridge University Press; 1996.

25 Hill M, Davis J, Prout A, Tinsdall K. Moving the participation agenda forward. *Child Soc*. 2004; **18**(2): 77–96.

26 Department of Health (DH). *Caring about Carers: a national strategy for carers*. London: DH; 1999. Available at: www.dh.gov.uk/en/Publicationsandstatistics/Publications/PublicationsPolicyAndGuidance/DH_4006522 (accessed 15 June 2010).

27 Frank J. *Making It Work: good practice with young carers and their families*. London: Children's Society; 2002.

28 Falkov A. *Crossing Bridges: training resources for working with mentally ill parents and their children*. London: Department of Health; 1998.

29 Walker O, Strong M, Atchinson R, *et al*. A qualitative study of primary care clinicians' views of treating childhood obesity. *BMC Fam Pract*. 2007; **8**: 1–6.

30 Princess Royal Trust for Carers. *Working with Young Carers*. London: Princess Royal Trust for Carers; 2009. Available at: www.carers.org/professionals/young-carers/ (accessed 15 June 2010).

31 Department of Health (DH). *Carers at the Heart of 21st Century Families and Communities*. London: DH; 2008.

32 Aldridge J. Picture this: the use of participatory photographic research methods with people with learning disabilities. *Disabil Soc*. 2007; **22**(1): 1–17.

33 Aldridge J, Sharpe, DM. *Pictures of Young Caring*. Loughborough: Young Carers Research Group, Loughborough University; 2007.

34 Hastings A. Assessing and improving the consultation skills of nurses. *Nurse Prescribing*. 2006; **4**(10): 418–22.

35 Radley A, Taylor D. Images of recovery: a photo elicitation study on the hospital ward. *Qual Health Res*. 2003; **13**(1): 77–99.

36 National Health Service (NHS) Information Centre. GPs spend longer with each patient as the number of consultations in general practice increases [Press release]. Available at: www.ic.nhs.uk/news-and-events/press-office/press-releases/archived-press-releases/april-2007--march-2008/gps-spend-longer-with-each-patient-as-the-number-of-consultations-in-general-practice-increases (accessed 15 June 2010).

37 Bernard P, Garralda ME, Hughes T. Evaluation of a teaching package in adolescent psychiatry for general practice registrars. *Educ Gen Prac*. 1999; **10**: 21–8.

38 See, for example, Highland Community Care Forum. *Connecting Young Carers*. 2009. Available at: www.highlandcommunitycareforum.org.uk/index.php?option=com_content&view=article&id=538&Itemid=262 (accessed 30 June 2010).

CHAPTER 7

Improving communication: practical exercises

Adrian Hastings

INTRODUCTION

In this chapter you will be told the stories of four children in the words used by the professionals they encounter, those of their parents or carers and the communication of the children themselves. Each story illuminates the concepts described in a preceding chapter to which it relates. They describe the opportunities that active listening offers to understand the child and the challenges that health professionals face in becoming truly expert at communication with children.

At intervals, as the story unfolds, you will be asked questions about your interpretation of what is being said (and perhaps as importantly what is being left unsaid), how you might act differently in the same situation and to reflect on how to improve your own skills. As a general practitioner, who has served the same community for 25 years, I continue to find ways of communicating better with the children I see. The four stories are fictional but they inevitably reflect the children and parents I have met as a GP. The community is largely white, working class with high levels of deprivation. Mothers are young, often poorly supported by the fathers of their children, although low levels of social mobility mean that the extended family is usually available to help.

1 INVOLVING CHILDREN: WHY IT MATTERS
Emma
Background

Emma Cranfield is 12 years old. She attends the nurse-led asthma clinic at her GP surgery. Her review is overdue and she cannot have more of her blue 'reliever' inhaler until she has been seen. The nurse observes from the medication record that she is not ordering brown 'preventer' inhalers. When considering what you would have done differently in each situation, refer back to Chapter 2, which discusses the importance of involving children.

Parental and professional factors

Nurse Sarah:	Good morning, Mrs Cranfield. Hello, Emma, is it really over a year since I saw you last? You've come for an asthma check today?
Mrs Cranfield:	Yes and I hope you can do something now. She's complaining about getting out of breath during games even though she uses her blue inhaler.
Nurse Sarah:	Does she use the brown inhaler?
Mrs Cranfield:	I don't like her using it – steroids are powerful drugs with a lot of bad side effects.
Nurse Sarah:	But you do have to use them if you need the blue inhaler every day. Could you check that she's doing so before breakfast and after supper?
Mrs Cranfield:	Maybe, but she's reaching puberty now and I don't want them to stunt her growth.
Nurse Sarah:	At the dose she is using that isn't going to be a problem. Do you understand how the different inhalers work?
Mrs Cranfield:	Yes, I've read the 'Parent's Guide to Asthma' you recommended last time but I think it is biased because it's sponsored by a drug company. It doesn't say anything about alternative therapies.

➤ What significant information have you noted?
➤ What good communication skills has the nurse used?
➤ What would you have done differently?

Commentary

Significant information

Emma's asthma is poorly controlled. Her mother has strong health beliefs and is informed about the potential risks of treatment. She has faith in alternative medicine so she may be colluding with Emma in her non-adherence to recommended treatment.

Good communication

Nurse Sarah has addressed Emma as well as her mother and by referring back to a previous consultation is developing a rapport. Her first question was directed to Emma. She is using conditional verbs (*'Could you'*) and she is checking understanding.

Alternative actions

I would try to involve Emma more: *'Hello, Emma, its nice to see you again. Good morning, Mrs Cranfield'*. The nurse then responded to the mother's statement about the effect of asthma on Emma with a question addressed to Mrs Cranfield, which caused the conversation to swing away from Emma. During the rest of the consultation she is referred to as 'she' and the adults talk over her head. As she is 12, the response to her mother's statement about being breathless during games should have been rephrased as, *'Do you use the brown inhaler Emma?'* In the exchange that follows the nurse could have said: *'But if you use the blue inhaler every day, as Emma does, then she needs to use the brown inhaler as well, before breakfast and after supper. You could do that, couldn't you, Emma?'*

It is important to know whether Emma's reason for not using the brown inhaler is the same as her mother's. The nurse has relied on a parental assessment of symptoms, rather than asking Emma to describe how her asthma affects her. At the age of 12, she is likely to have her own attitudes towards conventional and alternative medicine. These may concord with her mother's or she may be developing an independent viewpoint.

Promoting child involvement

Two weeks later Emma is seen by Dr Harrison in the Children's Assessment Unit because she has been brought to the hospital from school with difficulty in breathing. Her symptoms have improved with treatment and her mother is coming from work to take her home.

Dr Harrison:	Emma, how do you feel about having asthma?
Emma:	I hate it – I'm really good at hockey but I'll never get into the County Team when I get out of breath so much.
Dr Harrison:	Paul Scholes plays for 'Man U' and he's got asthma. How do you get on with your inhalers?
Emma:	I use them fine, the nurse checks up on me every time I go. If I need them at school I've got to go to the office and I know the teachers think I'm pulling a fast one.
Dr Harrison:	Which inhalers are you using?
Emma:	The blue and the brown, although Mum doesn't like me using the brown one much.
Dr Harrison:	Why is that? Doesn't she know the brown is the preventer?
Emma:	She wants me to use the Spongia pills from the homoeopathist. She says they are a natural remedy and they treat the cause not the symptoms.
Dr Harrison:	Homeopathy is rubbish! There's no evidence it works and it stops patients from getting the treatment they really need.
Emma:	I just wish my asthma would go away, it's ruining my life. I was supposed to be playing for the first team this afternoon.
Dr Harrison:	It doesn't have to be like that. Do you know why professional footballers with asthma are able to play at the top level? They take control of their treatment for themselves. They don't rely on others to do if for them.
Emma:	It's not like that for me! Everyone tells me what I should do but no one asks me what I think.

| Dr Harrison: | I'm sorry, you must think I am the same. I do understand why you feel like that – tell me what you think. |
| Emma: | If I believed the preventer inhaler really would work and isn't as bad as Mum says I'd use it more, like the nurse said. |

➤ What significant information have you noted?
➤ What good communication skills has the doctor used?
➤ What would you have done differently?

Commentary

Significant information

Playing hockey is very important to Emma and she sees her asthma as the main obstacle to success. She does not feel involved in decisions about her treatment and no one has explained to her the importance of correct use of preventer medication in treating asthma. She receives conflicting messages and her mother's negative attitudes are preventing adherence to treatment. The school's policy on restricting access to treatment via the office is further impeding Emma's ability to take full responsibility for her condition.

Good communication

Dr Harrison has made good use of the opportunity of talking to Emma without her mother present to explore why her asthma is poorly controlled. He started by asking about her feelings and explored her inhaler use with open questions. Even though he knew what medication she uses from seeing her earlier, he has created an opportunity to explore her adherence to treatment. By using examples relevant to her, he has been able to get her to realise that her asthma could be treated better. Emma's outburst sums up the pressure she is experiencing. Dr Harrison makes skilful use of an apology and an empathic statement to improve her trust of him.

Alternative actions

Dr Harrison ignores Emma's perceptions about the attitudes of her teachers. A simple response, such as *'Do they . . .?'*, would have given her an opportunity to elaborate. He asked a good open question, *'Why is that?'*, on learning about her mother's dislike of preventer inhalers. I would not have closed it down with a follow-up question, *'Doesn't she know the brown is the preventer?'*, as this assumes the answer and it is implicitly critical of Mrs Cranfield. He has allowed his strong beliefs about the ineffectiveness of homeopathy to add to Emma's sense that the adults around her have opinions that they want her to accept, rather than creating opportunities for her to explain her own thinking.

Child factors

Two months later Emma comes with her mother to the GP for a review of treatment of her asthma. While reviewing the record before the consultation Dr Kumar notes that she has missed an appointment for vaccination against cervical cancer two weeks ago. In listening to Emma's account she learns that her asthma has been much better since going to the hospital.

Dr Kumar:	I would like now to listen to your chest and do a breathing test. Can we go through into the examination room?
Dr Kumar:	I saw from the computer that you were due to come in two weeks ago for vaccination. [Pause] Did you get the appointment letter?
Emma:	The letter went to Mum. She told me about it but said she didn't believe it had been tested enough.
Dr Kumar:	Do you know the vaccination is to prevent cervical cancer?
Emma:	Yes, it said so in the letter. When we talked about it Mum said that you can have smear tests regularly to pick it up early so the vaccine isn't necessary. Even so, most of my friends have had it.
Dr Kumar:	You sound as if you wanted it.
Emma:	Well, Mum knows a lot about this sort of thing as she's always reading about health stuff, but I don't know.
Dr Kumar:	You don't know?
Emma:	It doesn't always work does it? The screening, I mean.
Dr Kumar:	Why do you say that?
Emma:	Julie's Mum has it bad – she's had chemo and been ill for months. I'd do anything not to have to go through that.
Dr Kumar:	Does anything mean having the vaccination?
Emma:	Yes, but I bet Mum won't let me – she thinks I'm not old enough to decide these things.
Dr Kumar:	Oh dear, I've put you in a bit of difficulty.

➤ What significant information have you noted?
➤ What good communication skills has the doctor used?
➤ What would you have done differently?

Commentary
Significant information

Mrs Cranfield believes that she remains the decision maker about healthcare matters affecting her 12-year-old daughter. She has chosen for her a preventive strategy, which is the one she uses herself. Emma's personal experience has been affected by seeing the mother of her friend suffering from cervical cancer and is now significantly different from Mrs Cranfield's.

Good communication

Dr Kumar's questions are open but focused. She signals to Emma that she wants to move to a completely different matter. By using silence she has allowed Emma to gather her thoughts. When she judges her to be ready she follows up with a question that does not assume an unwillingness to attend, which might have elicited a defensive response. She tests Emma's knowledge about the vaccine and by sensitivity to verbal cues (*'Even so, most of my friends have had it'*) is able to explore the gulf between Emma and her mother's priorities around vaccination.

Alternative actions

It is impossible to define at what age a child should take significant health decisions. Cognitive ability is a more important determinant. Dr Kumar recognised that it might have been difficult to explore the issue of vaccination in Mrs Cranfield's presence and therefore used the stratagem of taking Emma into an examination room to start the conversation. However, she herself is also in difficulty. Mrs Cranfield is likely to be resentful that Emma and the doctor have 'ganged up' on her. In this instance she would have done better to introduce the issue after fully dealing with the asthma review.

Some matters can be so sensitive it is necessary to talk to children on their own, having explained to their parents why you wish to do so. However, this is not one of them and a triadic approach to the issue of vaccination would have been more productive. She could have asked Emma who she thinks should be making healthcare decisions. Does Emma believe that she is capable to make decisions? What other decisions does she make in the rest of her life? Explain to Emma (and Mum) that by making decisions about one aspect of her care, she isn't expected to make all treatment choices and her Mum's input is still valued. Also explain to Emma that her Mum and the doctor can negotiate different courses of action to reduce any guilt or anxiety that she is somehow excluding her Mum, or deliberately going against her wishes.

2 INVOLVING CHILDREN: HOW TO DO IT

Shannon

Background

Shannon Newry is four years old. She has been referred to the hospital outpatient clinic by her GP because of abdominal pain and poor weight gain. She is to see Dr Wilson, a paediatrician with an interest in gastroenterology. Dr Johnson is a first-year specialist registrar and has been asked to make the initial assessment. She enters the clinic room and sees three people: a middle-aged woman, rather untidily dressed in a loose-fitting jumper and slacks, sitting next to a pretty girl who looks to be around 11 years old, in a pink tee shirt and black leggings, and Shannon, who is sitting on the floor, looking at a book with her back to the door.

How would you start the consultation? You could refer back to Chapter 4, which describes a model of the consultation. The first two steps are to interpret the information known about the patient before the consultation starts and to set your goals.

Opening the consultation

Dr Johnson: Hello, Shannon, I'm Dr Johnson. How are you today?
Shannon: [Carries on looking at her book.]
Dr Johnson: OK, I'll just have a word with your Mum.

Doreen:	I'm her Nan. Maxine's at work so she asked me to bring Shannon to get her sorted out.
Dr Johnson:	Can you tell me more about the problem?
Doreen:	Maxine's fed up with it. Shannon's always getting pains in the tummy. She picks at her food and the health visitor says she's underweight. All the doctor did was give her Calpol and a diet sheet when Maxine took her – he didn't even examine her. When she went back a month later to say it wasn't working he said he didn't know what was wrong and that you would find out.
Dr Johnson:	Do you know why he didn't examine her?

➤ What significant information have you noted?
➤ What good communication skills has the doctor used?
➤ What would you have done differently?

Commentary

Significant information

The family are probably economically deprived. Shannon is relaxed but perhaps not interested in why she is here. The other child is likely to be a sibling and their relationship may be relevant. Her mother might be a single-parent in a low-paid job. People in professional occupations have more flexibility in their work schedules and can afford to take time out. Maxine has the support of her extended family. The phrase *'get her sorted out'* implies that Shannon is seen as the source of a problem. There is an implicit criticism of the actions of the GP.

Good communication

Dr Johnson started by addressing Shannon and introducing herself. She went on to use an open question of Doreen to discover the main presenting problems.

Alternative actions

First ensure everyone is seated in a suitable arrangement before starting. At age four, sitting on Nan's lap is usually the best position for Shannon. I would make eye contact with everyone in the room and open with a non-clinical topic. *'How are you today?'* is not a suitable opening for a four-year-old. Young children will often converse comfortably with adults who are strangers through a shared object, such as a toy or book, chatting about one or two of the pictures.

It would help to know everyone's preference for address. Children expect adults will use their first names when talking to them. I address adults by their title and surname and expect them to use my title and surname. Other doctors are comfortable to be on first-name terms with patients, but this introduces imbalance when working with children, as very few would address a doctor by a first name. A good compromise is to use your title and first name (e.g. Dr Emily). Once the introductions have been made and Shannon had been reassured by the chat about her book it would be a good time to ask her if she knows why she has come.

The statement, *'Maxine's fed up with it'*, is covert criticism of Shannon, which, at the age of four, she would probably understand. Dr Johnson should note this and plan how to help Shannon feel less demeaned by it. As reported, the GP has performed poorly. However, this is a second-hand account and Dr Johnson's response could be interpreted as agreeing with Maxine's criticism. It would have been better to respond to the positive statement and say, *'that is what we are here for; tell me more about Shannon's problem'*.

Gathering information

Dr Johnson:	Whereabouts does Shannon get the pain?
Doreen:	It can be all over but it's mainly on the left, especially if she's trying to poo.
Dr Johnson:	What kind of pain is it?
Doreen:	It can be really bad – it even wakes her up at night.
Dr Johnson:	When did it start?
Doreen:	She's had it on and off for over a year.
Dr Johnson:	Does anything make it better or worse?
Doreen:	Not really. We've tried putting a hot-water bottle on her tummy and rubbing it but it just seems to take its time to go.
Dr Johnson:	Is it worse when she has something to eat?
Doreen:	I don't think so.
Dr Johnson:	Does she have any diarrhoea?
Doreen:	Yes, and that's the worst of it. She's often messing her pants. She's started hiding them under her bed in case Maxine gives her a smack.
Dr Johnson:	You mustn't smack children who soil themselves – it makes the problem worse.

➤ What significant information have you noted?
➤ What good communication skills has the doctor used?
➤ What would you have done differently?

Commentary

Significant information

Through her questions Dr Johnson has elicited more information about the problem of 'tummy pains', although further detail will need to be sought before a provisional list of differential diagnoses can be constructed. There is an additional significant problem, not mentioned initially, of faecal incontinence that will require further exploration.

Good communication

The doctor has used simple, clear language in her questions and these have been mainly straightforward.

Alternative actions

At this stage, it is essential to involve Shannon in the consultation. This will allow an assessment of her developmental stage, social skills and feelings to be initiated. At the age of four she is likely to be reserved with strangers and may be fearful of health professionals. If she has normal linguistic development she will have a large vocabulary for things she has experienced but a limited understanding of abstract concepts (e.g. she will understand objects can be hot or cold but not that they have a temperature). I would direct my enquiry about the pain to Shannon but be aware that she is still at an age when she is suggestible and will tend to respond 'yes' to most questions, therefore a simple, open-question style may be needed.

Dr Johnson has failed to elicit anything about the timing of the tummy pain other than when it began. Knowing about the frequency and duration of the episodes of pain, whether they happen at particular times of day and whether the problem is progressing, is essential in problem solving the possible diagnostic causes. She has also asked one double question, *'Does anything make it better or worse?'* As a result she is told about actions that do not relieve the pain but has to repeat the question about what does makes it worse. Her response, *'You mustn't smack . . .'*, could have used the pronoun 'we', as this is less directly critical and helps the group to share the problem. Dr Johnson's concern about Maxine's response to incontinence has led her prematurely into the management phase of the consultation. She is giving the patient advice about what she needs to do to tackle the problem before she has made her own diagnosis, much less achieved a shared understanding of the problem. I would make a mental note that I will need to explore the family's ideas, concerns and understanding of incontinence in children once I judge that I have developed sufficient rapport for Shannon and her Nan to trust me.

Exploring the impact of the problem

Dr Johnson:	What do you think is causing Shannon's tummy problem?
Doreen:	I think she's attention seeking. I know Maxine has to work, what with two of them to bring up on her own, but I don't hold with that when they are little. They need their Mum around.
Dr Johnson:	Why do you think that?
Doreen:	The girls in the nursery are hardly more than children themselves. They don't know Shannon like we do.
Dr Johnson:	Sorry, I meant why do you think she's attention seeking?
Doreen:	She's a bit of a madam. When she was younger she used to have screaming fits in the supermarket if she didn't get any sweets. It's not her fault she's like it 'cos Maxine's out so much but she can be a real handful.
Shannon:	[Wriggles off Doreen's lap and goes over to where the older child is texting on her mobile phone.]
Dr Johnson:	Do you know what Maxine's worried about?
Doreen:	She's starting school full-time soon; the children and teachers

	will know if she has an accident. The school might even send her home.
Dr Johnson:	What's her diet like?
Doreen:	She's very picky with her food; there's so many things she won't eat and then she wants crisps and biscuits because she's hungry.
Leanne:	Mum went mad at her last night.

➤ What significant information have you noted?
➤ What good communication skills has the doctor used?
➤ What would you have done differently?

Commentary

Significant information

Our assumption that Maxine is a single parent has been confirmed. Despite Doreen's apparent support to Maxine there may be important differences of opinion about parenting between them. Doreen may think that Maxine gives in too easily to Shannon's demands. There is concern that the problem of abdominal pain and faecal incontinence might interfere with Shannon's schooling, even leading to bullying. Maxine may be worried that her job will be at risk if she is called by the school. Shannon appears to have learnt that she can manipulate her mother into giving her preferred foods by refusing to eat prepared meals. Leanne's contribution indicates that Maxine may feel under considerable pressure to adhere to previous advice about diet and that the problem is causing her emotions to become out of control.

Good communication

Dr Johnson is using open questions, attempting to gain a better impression of the impact of the problem on the family. By avoiding closed questions at this stage she is signalling to Doreen that she is interested to learn their views. She is exploring the family's ideas, concerns and expectations and in the process has gained important additional information about the psychological and social issues affecting the family.

Alternative actions

The exchange between Doreen and Dr Johnson is resulting in a negative impression of Shannon in which she is cast as a 'problem child'. Although children often appear not to be heeding the discourse between adults they usually listen with more care than we assume. When talking with the adult it is important to observe the child's body language to assess the impact of the conversation. There is evidence that Shannon dislikes what Doreen and Dr Johnson are discussing by distancing herself from them. Leanne too has been listening carefully and her intervention is exquisitely timed to have maximum effect on the adults. Every consultation contains a wealth of verbal and non-verbal cues available to the health professional taking it. By developing the skills of recognising these, interpreting their meanings and then exploring them with children and their carers you will become much more effective in your work. As soon as the pejorative term *attention seeking* was used I would consider ways of enabling Shannon's voice to be heard. Dr Johnson could now make eye contact with Shannon, smile at her and quietly ask her one or two general questions about home or school, before going on to ask, *'What do you think is wrong with your tummy?'* This signals that she is interested in Shannon and values her views. Of course, Shannon may refuse to say anything and answering the question literally requires a level of knowledge and abstraction beyond the capability of a four-year-old. However, the manner of asking it and the use of the words 'you' and 'your' to Shannon show that it is safe for her to respond.

Examination

Dr Johnson:	Shannon, if I am going to help you with your tummy I need to have a look at it.
Shannon:	[Appears apprehensive and pulls the hem of her tee shirt down.]
Dr Johnson:	My Teddy has a poorly tummy; will you help me make him better?
Shannon:	[Lets go of her tee shirt and peers round Dr Johnson's back to see the teddy she is holding.]
Dr Johnson:	I'll put him on the desk and we can look at him together.
Dr Johnson:	[Involves Shannon in looking at Teddy's tummy, gently feeling it and then listening to it with a stethoscope]
Dr Johnson:	Can I look at yours now?
Shannon:	No.
Dr Johnson:	It won't hurt and I can't make you better unless you let me do it.
Shannon:	Don't want to. Don't like it.

➤ What significant information have you noted?
➤ What good communication skills has the doctor used?
➤ What would you have done differently?

Commentary
Significant information

Shannon has a normal level of understanding for her age and has now relaxed enough with Dr Johnson to participate in the game of examining Teddy's tummy. However, she is still anxious about being touched by the doctor. This may signify a previous unpleasant experience, possibly involving a rectal examination by her GP.

Good communication

Dr Johnson started with an affirmative statement and quickly picked up the cue. She responded by showing Shannon what she was going to do using the teddy as a model, rather than telling her in words.

Alternative actions

The opening statement could have been replaced with the game of examining Teddy. *'My Teddy has a poorly tummy. Let's see if we can make him better'*. Ascertaining from Shannon why she is anxious about the examination is essential. If the abdominal examination is going to reveal findings (positive or negative) that are important in making a diagnosis, then doing it is not an option that Shannon can accept or refuse. A direct question, *'Can I look at yours now?'*, often elicits a negative response. During the teddy game more time could be spent with all three participants taking turns. *'Feel Teddy's tummy Shannon. Is it soft? Now you feel your tummy. Is it soft like Teddy's?'* Even Teddy can get a turn using the stethoscope to listen to Shannon's tummy, for example.

Dr Johnson has assumed that Shannon's reluctance is out of fear of pain but using the words, *'It won't hurt'*, may have the paradoxical effect of making her more resistant. It would be better to extend the game she played with Teddy by using one of the techniques mentioned in Chapter 4, such as, *'I'm going to guess what you had for breakfast!'* Sometimes it is unavoidable to do an examination or other procedure that is unpleasant or painful. Dr Johnson will need to be sure that a rectal examination will provide key information – if this is the case then she should postpone it until she has completed all other elements of the history and examination. Before doing the examination Dr Johnson must say exactly what she is going to do.

Management

Dr Johnson has discussed her assessment of Shannon's problem with Dr Wilson and they have agreed that the diagnosis is chronic constipation, with faecal incontinence due to overflow diarrhoea.

Dr Wilson:	Hello, Shannon, I'm Dr Emily. Who has come with you today?
Shannon:	Me Nan and Leanne.
Dr Wilson:	Hello, Leanne, are you Shannon's sister?
Leanne:	Yes, and I help Mum look after her. I'm in Year 6 now!
Dr Wilson:	Well, you've all come today so we can help Shannon with her tummy problem. I need to know a bit more about the food you like to eat at home. Shannon, what did you have for breakfast?
Shannon:	[Looks round at Nan but does not answer.]
Dr Wilson:	Leanne, can you help?
Leanne:	I had Weetabix and toast but Shannon only likes Coco Pops.
Dr Wilson:	What did you have for tea last night?
Leanne:	Mum did us sausage and mash with carrots, and banana custard for afters.
Dr Wilson:	That sounds lovely. Did you eat it all?
Leanne:	I did but Shannon only had the mash. In the end Mum gave her chocolate ice cream 'cos she said she was still hungry.
Dr Wilson:	I think your Mum's good at cooking. [Smiles and catches Nan's eye] We need to write down a list of meals for you for the whole week. You see Shannon's tummy problem will only get better when she has the right things to eat.

➤ What significant information have you noted?
➤ What good communication skills has the doctor used?
➤ What would you have done differently?

Commentary

Significant information

The age gap of six or seven years between the sisters has meant that Leanne sees herself as having some 'parental' responsibility. The food that Maxine is providing is varied and healthy, with a reasonable content of dietary fibre. However, Shannon is choosing to eat the foods with least fibre, which is contributing to her constipation.

Good communication

Dr Wilson has addressed Shannon first and invited her to make the introductions. This makes her the focus of attention and gives her a straightforward task to accomplish. She greets Leanne and invites her to contribute when Shannon chooses not to answer her question. She uses inclusive language, *'we can help . . .'*, and, *'we need to . . .'*, to indicate shared ownership of the problem and its solution. She is making positive affirmations about the absent Maxine and, through non-verbal communication, is indicating to Nan that her contributions will be sought in due course.

Alternative actions

Dr Wilson has started to provide the family with advice on what to do. It may be that Dr Johnson has already explained the diagnosis to them; even so Dr Wilson should take the opportunity to go over it again. It will be important to involve Shannon in discussion of the management using appropriate language and reinforcing this with pictures of which food is best and how the body makes 'poo'. Reaching a shared understanding of overflow incontinence with them herself will allow her to check their beliefs and their readiness to cooperate with the complex plan needed for successful resolution of the problem.

3 PROFESSIONAL SPEAK AND CHILD TALK

Wayne

Background

Wayne is two years old. He is the youngest of Pat Marriott's four children. His sisters, who are aged 16, 14 and 13, have a different father. Wayne's father, Sean Morton, lives with the family. He works intermittently as a general labourer on building sites. As you read the account of Wayne's life over a year you will be asked at intervals to consider the evidence for poor interprofessional working that his story reveals and suggest how an alternative approach would have produced a better outcome. Chapter 5 describes the roles and skills of the different health and social care professionals responsible for children and indicates how good interprofessional working is essential to deliver effective care to them.

At the hospital

Wayne was born with a talipes equinovarus (club foot) deformity of his left ankle. His mother has not been able to adhere to the Ponseti Method of serial casting; she has missed follow-up appointments and it has been decided he will require surgery to correct the deformity. The nurse who admits him to the ward the night before his operation records:

> *Head lice on admission, hair washed with Lyclear. No change of clothes to go home in after surgery. Cried on and off during the night, asking for Mummy.*

The operation goes well and he is discharged later that day. His mother is given a letter to deliver to her GP surgery, which is copied and sent to his health visitor by post. The letter states:

> *Anterior tibial tendon transfer. ROS seven days. Ibuprofen as needed for pain relief. See in clinic in 4 weeks.*

Evidence for poor interprofessional working

The nurse has made a clear record of her observations. These suggest that Wayne's mother has difficulty in providing him with an appropriate standard of care. However, the discharge summary report which was prepared by the specialist trainee registrar (STR) simply gives information about the medical procedure. This will be the only written communication that the hospital provides to members of the primary care team as full, dictated discharge summary letters have been replaced by standardised forms completed at a computer station. It is rare for medical staff to review the nursing records when they see patients on the ward.

Alternative approach

The nurse could have shared her concerns with the STR. However, shift patterns of work for doctors in training have reduced the opportunities for individual professionals on a ward to meet informally and discuss their patients. Some doctors see their role as restricted to providing good care for the specific disease they are qualified to treat and would regard other issues as the preserve of others to manage. If the doctor had such attitudes, the nurse might feel inhibited in raising her concerns with him. The nurse could have rung Wayne's health visitor or written a note to her. She might be deterred from these actions by uncertainty about how the health visitor will respond. A clumsy approach by the health visitor could anger the mother, even to the point of making a complaint that the nurse has made a prejudicial judgement about her parenting skills without discussing her concerns directly with her.

GP surgery

Eight weeks later Wayne is brought to his GP with an earache. Before the consultation starts, Dr Alton observes that there is a letter in Wayne's record, received the previous week:

General Hospital Paediatric Physiotherapy Clinic. Did not attend. In line with Trust policy has been discharged. If still in need of treatment a new referral will be required.

After advising on the treatment of an ear infection the GP asks why Wayne did not attend for physiotherapy.

Mrs Marriott:	Lisa came home really late the night before, there was a big row and I forgot the next day that I should have gone to the hospital.
Dr Alton:	You do need to let them know if you can't make it. Now they've discharged Wayne I'll have to write them another letter. Please, make sure you keep the appointment this time.
Mrs Marriott:	I'm so sorry doctor, there's so much going off at the moment. Wayne's not been sleeping properly since the operation, Lisa's being really difficult about school and Sean's not helping much now he's back in work.
Dr Alton:	Who's your health visitor – can't she arrange some help for you?
Mrs Marriott:	Since they moved out to the Children's Centre I've not seen her.
Dr Alton:	I've lost track of who's who these days. I'll send an email message to reception now to get someone from the Children's Centre to give you a ring.

Dr Alton types the following message immediately after the consultation:

> *Please ring Children's Centre and ask health visitor to get in touch with Mrs Marriott. She has missed hospital appointments for follow-up after Wayne's operation and is struggling with teenage daughter, who seems to be off the rails at the moment.*

Evidence for poor interprofessional working

The physiotherapy department has made no attempt to establish the reasons for Wayne's non-attendance. While missed appointments cause substantial disruption for health services it is not proper for children to miss essential treatment because of parental disorganisation. There is no guarantee that the GP will act on receiving the letter. Unless the GP who reads it knows Wayne and his family, he is likely to send it to be filed, awaiting a future attendance. Communication of this nature is prone to irritate the GP, who will regard the task of writing another letter as a bureaucratic imposition by the hospital.

Dr Alton's understandable annoyance with the hospital has coloured his communication with Mrs Marriott and she now feels guilty about the missed appointment. She has provided important information about problems within the family but he is not now receptive to these and is seeking to delegate the task of assessing them to a colleague. His frustration with poorly functioning systems has caused him to make a statement that is implicitly critical of the health visiting service. Fragmentation of traditional patterns of working between members of the primary care team caring for children under five means that effective communication between them happens less than it used to. Familiarity with individual colleagues has been reduced and impersonal methods of communication have replaced conversations.

Alternative approach

A telephone call to Mrs Marriott that day, after the missed appointment, would have discovered why she did not come, and that she was still willing to bring Wayne for treatment. This would have taken the physiotherapist substantially less time than she would have spent in providing the treatment. It also has the potential of identifying significant needs that are preventing Wayne's adherence to treatment.

Every consultation offers many more opportunities for promoting good health than can be acted on. It is a challenge to prioritise these appropriately. Dr Alton could have briefly explored with Mrs Marriott in what way Lisa is being difficult about school. An awareness of the roles of other professionals such as the school nurse and school counsellor would allow him to suggest an effective source of help that Mrs Marriott could access, without this taking an excessive amount of time.

Speech and language therapy

Wayne's health visitor had previously noted that he had a restricted vocabulary two months before his second birthday. She referred him to the speech therapist and after a four-month delay he is attending for an assessment.

Ms Eastwood:	You may think I've just been playing with Wayne for the last half-hour but in fact I have been taking note of what he has been saying and how he is using words. I must say he is behind where he should be for a child of his age.
Mrs Marriott:	I don't know about that. The girls were quicker than him but Jodie had the same problem with her lad and she was told boys are slower to talk than girls.
Ms Eastwood:	How much time are you able to spend talking with him?
Mrs Marriott:	I do what I can – but there's a lot to do. As well as looking after the house I have a cleaning job at the school from four 'til seven.
Ms Eastwood:	Do you have the TV on during the day?
Mrs Marriott:	Oh yes! He loves *In the Night Garden* – it really keeps him quiet. I think he learns a lot from it. He knows all their names and where they live.
Ms Eastwood:	Who looks after him when you are at work?
Mrs Marriott:	The girls do. At least one of them gets home before I have to go

to work. They're hooked on *Deal or No Deal* so he sits with them while they watch. I leave the tea made up and they feed Wayne while they're watching telly and put him to bed after.

Ms Eastwood: Is he a good sleeper?

Mrs Marriott: Not really; he often wakes up in the middle of the night wanting something to eat so I have to give him a Kit Kat.

Ms Eastwood: Does he not eat properly during the day?

Mrs Marriott: He's so picky about his food and takes ages to eat so I think the girls get a bit bored feeding him and that's why he's hungry.

Ms Eastwood prepares a detailed report of her assessment. A copy of this is sent to Wayne's health visitor and general practitioner. On the fourth page in her conclusion she writes:

> *Wayne's language development is poor for his age. I think this is largely because his family does not converse with him as much as required. I was not able to detect any specific condition causing delay in language acquisition. I have therefore advised his mother about techniques to encourage him to lead conversations, giving him time to speak and to use mapping to scaffold word development. Incidentally, I thought he was rather thin so I suggested to his mother that his weight should be checked. Although any failure to gain weight is likely to be secondary to the family's culture around food he may require referral for investigation of failure to thrive.*

Evidence for poor interprofessional working

The speech therapist has learnt some very important facts about how the Marriott family functions. Wayne's poor language development is probably due to him having few meaningful conversations with adults in the day. He is a passive recipient of verbal communication that is detached from the world he inhabits. His mother is experiencing substantial pressure managing her different roles as parent, partner and worker. Wayne is receiving care from teenage sisters at one of the most important times of the day for social interaction and development. Multiple distractions at tea time are preventing him from eating sufficient food and he is 'topping up' in the night with a chocolate biscuit.

Although this picture is alluded to in Ms Eastwood's report the detailed, nuanced information does not come through. Her specific recommendation about scaffolding assumes a level of understanding of what this requires that the GP and the health visitor may not possess, so they will be unable to explain and encourage Mrs Marriott to use it. Having picked up the potentially serious problem of failure to thrive her suggestion for how this should be followed up is vague. It would be easy for both the GP and the health visitor to assume the other will do so. Moreover, the most important part of her lengthy report is hidden at the end. Reports of this nature are primarily a legible summary in the records of the team that generates them, to which they can refer back on future occasions. Communication with colleagues from different teams is a secondary purpose.

Alternative approach

It is necessary for all health professionals to remember that the jargon of their profession is not inevitably understood by others. Even within the same profession different disciplines use terminology that is unfamiliar to non-specialists. Therefore a term such as 'mapping to scaffold' should be explained in explicit terms so that the GP and health visitor can help the mother to implement this technique.

GPs will receive around 30 items of written communication each day, with an average of 500 words or numbers in each one. Inevitably, the majority of these are skimmed to extract the key items of information. It is much more likely that important steps are taken if the report starts with a list of these, preferably highlighted in some way. If a recommendation for action is required it should be accompanied by a clear statement from the author about how this should be achieved and who is responsible for doing it.

At the Children's Centre

Mrs Marriott has brought Wayne to the 'Messy Play' session on Saturday morning. During the snack break she speaks to one of the nursery nurses.

Mrs Marriott:	When he went to speech therapy the lady said I ought to get him weighed. Could you do it for me now to save me coming back in the week?
Jenny Elston:	Yes, of course, have you got the Red Book* with you?
Mrs Marriott:	Oh, sorry. I left it at home, but I can remember what he weighed last time. He was exactly 24 pounds then.
Jenny Elston:	[Stands him on the scales and reads his weight] He's 12 kilos today.
Mrs Marriott:	How much is that in pounds?
Jenny Elston:	Let me see, I've got the chart here. Yes, over 26, nearly 27 pounds so that means he's put on about three pounds.
Mrs Marriott:	That doesn't sound too bad.
Jenny Elston:	Well, it's important to get him weighed regularly so make sure you bring in the Red Book next time and we'll write it down and put it on the chart.

Evidence for poor interprofessional working

Jenny Elston has been flexible and helpful to Mrs Marriott even though she probably has procedures to follow that would instruct her to bring Wayne back on another occasion. She has demonstrated awareness of the importance of being opportunistic in health promotion when families do not adhere to established routines. However, she has inadvertently reassured Mrs Marriott that Wayne's growth is satisfactory

---

*   A colloquial term for the Child Health Record for under-fives which contains records of all developmental assessments, immunisations and monitoring of growth using percentile charts.

because she has not established the interval between the two weights. As the first was done when he was 18 months and this one at the age of 30 months he has in fact moved from the 25th percentile weight for age to the 10th. This means that he may be failing to thrive.

Alternative approach

It is possible that she is acting beyond her level of competence in weighing Wayne and that she should have sought advice from a more experienced colleague before doing so. If this was not available to her at the time, it is necessary to communicate the weight recorded today to the health visitor and the GP in writing.

Conclusion

Chapter 5 describes what each profession has to offer children in supporting them to reach their full potential for good health and development. Chapter 9 describes the consequences for them when poor or malicious parenting meets with professional incompetence, especially expressed as ineffective communication with colleagues. The message from these chapters and Wayne's story is that colleagues from other professions have skills, which children require, that we do not possess. Joint working requires we recognise this truth. The modern working environment often curtails good team-working practice as opportunities for the most important form of communication – face-to-face – have been reduced. Respect for the roles of other professions will reduce harmful conflict and enable more effective collaboration. If it is not possible to meet with a colleague a telephone conversation (properly noted in the record) is the next most effective method of communication as it allows for checking and negotiation. When this is not possible it is necessary for written communications to be unambiguous, specific and correctly directed.

4 LISTENING TO YOUNG CARERS AND THEIR FAMILIES
Abbie
Background

Abbie is 10 years old. She attends more frequently than is usual at her GP surgery with a variety of minor illnesses. She is seeing the doctor on an emergency appointment in the afternoon surgery with her mother, Justine. After establishing that she has been off school for the last week with an upper respiratory tract infection the GP asks what her mother was expecting from the consultation. As you read the account of her meetings with health and education professionals revisit Chapter 6, which describes the particular needs of children who are caring for adults.

Duality and tensions

Justine: I rang the school today to say Abbie wouldn't be in because she's got a bad cold. They said I have to get a note from the doctor as she's missed too much school this term.

Dr Evans: We don't usually do certificates for schools – and when we do

	we have to charge for them.
Justine:	I can't afford to pay, I'm a single parent and I'm not working.
Dr Evans:	You can take an appointment slip to show them you've been to the doctor – there's no charge for that.
Justine:	You tell him, Abbie. They're always on to us about you having time off.
Dr Evans:	Is that true, Abbie? Are you having trouble at school?
Abbie:	No, I like school but I can't always go and they think I am bunking off.
Dr Evans:	Well, you have come here to see us a few times this year. Mum would you like me to talk to Abbie's teacher?
Justine:	Yes, Doctor, anything to stop them hassling us.

➤ What significant information have you noted?
➤ What good communication skills has the doctor used?
➤ What would you have done differently?

Commentary
Significant information
It is probable that Abbie has missed an unwarrantable amount of school lately. Her poor attendance is unlikely to be school refusal as she says she likes going. There is therefore another reason. Justine is reporting significant social stress factors. She is imposing unjustifiable pressure on her daughter by telling her to explain to the doctor. Her use of the terms *'they'* and *'us'* in this context and the word *'hassling'* indicate that she feels the world is against them.

Good communication
The doctor is able to negotiate an alternative to payment for a private certificate. She asks for permission to talk to the teacher and in a way that allows Justine to dissent if she wishes.

Alternative actions
I would have clarified what Justine meant by saying 'too much school' before explaining my reluctance to issue a certificate. Dr Evans asks Abbie if her mother has been truthful which risks offending Justine. She makes an assumption that her poor attendance is because of problems at school rather than inviting her to explain why she has not been going. She does not pick up the cue, *'I can't always go'*, which is a missed opportunity to explore her attitudes to school.

Referral and multi-agency collaboration
Dr Evans reviews Abbie's full record, which does not reveal any reason for her missing school other than minor illness. She is unfamiliar with the family so she looks for the records of other members of the household. Justine is the only person registered with the practice. She is an insulin-dependent diabetic, whose blood sugar control is poor.

She rings the school to speak to Abbie's class teacher, Mrs Williams, who confirms she has been absent for a third of school days in the last year. Furthermore, Justine sometimes appears inebriated when collecting Abbie in the afternoon. Dr Evans asks Mrs Williams if she can find out more next time Abbie is at school.

Mrs Williams:	Abbie, you went to see Dr Evans last week, what did she say?
Abbie:	That she'd talk to you about me missing school.
Mrs Williams:	Yes, she did but she told me you'd not had any serious illness. [Pause]
Abbie:	Well, I've had lots of colds this winter and Mum says I'll pick up another if I come back too soon.
Mrs Williams:	Why does she say that?
Abbie:	I dunno.
Mrs Williams:	Last month you came to school late three days in one week, and I know you didn't have a cold then.
Abbie:	I overslept – we haven't got an alarm.
Mrs Williams:	Is there any other reason?
Abbie:	No, not really.
Mrs Williams:	Not really?
Abbie:	If I say, you won't tell anyone, will you?
Mrs Williams:	What is it, that I would tell them?
Abbie:	I can't say.
Mrs Williams:	Abbie, I want to help you. If you trust me I promise I won't talk to anyone unless you say I can.
Abbie:	Mum often needs me to give her insulin injections.
Mrs Williams:	Why is that?
Abbie:	'Cos her hand shakes too much to draw up the right number of units.
Mrs Williams:	Has anyone talked to you about giving your Mum her insulin injections?
Abbie:	No, I don't need to, Mum's shown me what to do and besides I'm afraid what they'll do if they know.
Mrs Williams:	What do you think they'll do?
Abbie:	Mum says they could put me into care.
Mrs Williams:	They won't do that.
Abbie:	It happened before when I was four.
Mrs Williams:	I'm sorry about that. Will you tell me what happened last month when you were late?
Abbie:	Like I said, Mum couldn't give herself the insulin.
Mrs Williams:	You said her hands were shaking too much. Do you know why they do that?
Abbie:	It's always after she's been late at the club. She has too much to drink and she gets up late, and is hung over.
Mrs Williams:	Abbie, I think we need to help you and your Mum. Will you let me talk to Dr Evans? Then I will see you again and chat to you

about what's been happening.

Commentary

Significant information

The stated reasons for missing school are not consistent. Abbie is expected to perform a potentially hazardous task for her mother, as an incorrect dose of insulin could be very harmful. Abbie and Justine fear that professional intervention in their situation could lead to the break-up of the family and are not willing to disclose her caring role. The report from the school and Abbie's account suggest that Justine's misuse of alcohol is at a dangerous level and that she and Abbie are at significant risk of harm.

Good communication

Mrs Williams consistently explores Abbie's thoughts and feelings using open questions, silence and prompts to continue (*'Not really?'*). When the question to explore Justine's health beliefs around colds is unsuccessful she uses an alternative approach to probe. She recognises when a statement is concealing the truth and explores further without challenging the implausible explanation, *'We haven't got an alarm'*. She explains that the motivation for her questions is to help Abbie and asks for her trust and permission for the actions she will take.

Alternative actions

I would be wary of giving commitments about confidentiality until I was sure that I could honour these. Mrs Williams promises *'not to talk to anyone'* at a point in the interview when she may later hear something that obliges her to act without Abbie's consent. In attempting to reassure Abbie (*'They won't do that'*) she risks losing all of the trust she is seeking to develop by stating something that Abbie's own experience tells her is incorrect.

Support to relinquish responsibilities

Dr Evans and Mrs Williams discuss the situation over the phone and concur that there are substantial grounds for believing Abbie to be at risk of serious harm, as well as the actual damage from the disruption of her education. They agree that the school will take responsibility and implement its child protection policy. This states that the person with nominated responsibility should investigate further and report to the Social Services Department. Mrs Williams arranges for Justine and Abbie to come to a meeting with the head teacher, Mrs Dauncey. After establishing that Mrs Williams has gained an accurate picture of the situation she seeks to ascertain Abbie's wishes about possible solutions.

Mrs Dauncey:	Abbie, how do you feel about giving insulin injections to your Mum?
Abbie:	Well, I've got to do it, haven't I? I've seen what happens to her when she has to go to hospital. I don't want that to happen again.

Mrs Dauncey:	Who looked after you then?
Abbie:	Me Auntie Sharan. She lives the other side of the Tic Toc Park.
Mrs Dauncey:	Do you like staying with her?
Abbie:	Yes, I get to play with Andy and Skye and go on the Internet on their computer.
Mrs Dauncey:	I can tell you don't like giving the injections. Am I right?
Abbie:	Yes, I don't like giving her injections, but after she comes back from the club she is drunk. I hate that!
Mrs Dauncey:	Would you like to go and live with your Auntie until your Mum is well again?
Abbie:	No, I just want Mum to stop drinking so much. If I went away, she'd be worse.
Mrs Dauncey:	Justine, what do you think?
Justine:	Abbie's right, I'm so stupid, I try not to go out but some nights I just need to get away from the house and meet people. The club's the only place to go and once I get a drink down me I can't seem to stop.
Mrs Dauncey:	Do you worry about her being in the house on her own?
Justine:	I do afterwards, but she's so grown up for her age I know she can manage. I take my mobile and if she phones me I always come home straight away.
Mrs Dauncey:	Abbie, how do you feel when you are in the house on your own?
Abbie:	I'm not scared 'cos I know Buster will frighten any burglars away and Mum does always come home if I ring, but I just know she'll be ill in the morning and that makes me feel sad.
Mrs Dauncey:	Abbie, we are concerned that it's not safe for you as things are. We do need to get help for you and your Mum. Do you understand why we have to ask the Social Services to look into what's happening?
Abbie:	I don't want to leave Mum but I do want her to stop drinking. If they can do that then it's ok with me.

➤ What significant information have you noted?
➤ What good communication skills has the head teacher used?
➤ What would you have done differently?

Commentary

Significant information

Justine has had serious complications of her diabetes in the past and Abbie feels responsible for preventing these in the future. There is potential support to the family from Justine's sister. Abbie is distressed by her mother's drunkenness and does not want the responsibility of giving insulin. Justine has a serious problem of alcohol abuse and an unrealistic view of the capability of Abbie to act in the carer's role. She has considerable health and social care needs that will require intensive support if the family is to remain together.

Good communication

Mrs Dauncey uses Abbie's name at every opportunity. Together with her clear, open questions this ensures that the interview is consistently focused on exploring Abbie's feelings and opinions. She avoids a confrontational approach with her mother, which would be likely to elicit an unproductive, defensive response, perhaps intensified by the guilt Justine feels about the demands she is making of Abbie. She recognises that she is obliged to report this situation to Social Services so does not pretend this is an optional decision. In stating this she leads in by expressing concern for Abbie's safety and that the motivation is to help her and Justine.

Alternative actions

Although I may have approached this interview differently because of my clinical background, there are no suggestions for improvement I would make to Mrs Dauncey about her questions and statements. Now that the full picture has been brought into the open the school is responsible for ensuring effective communication about the situation and the needs of both Justine and Abbie to those who are able to provide support. This will require awareness of the different referral pathways.

CHAPTER 8

Consent and confidentiality

Anne Willmott

INTRODUCTION

Dealing with children and young people can bring a number of potential dilemmas. What do I do if a 15-year-old refuses a test or treatment? Can I treat a child if the parents aren't there? What happens if a young person tells me something in confidence that I need to share? In all of our dealings with children we need to be aware of, and work within, what the law and national guidance require of us. Clearly an exhaustive review of this topic is outside the scope of this book, but in this chapter we will first consider terms used in relation to consulting with children (such as parental responsibility and 'Gillick competence'), and current legislation on consent, refusal of consent and the treatment of an unaccompanied child. Finally, we will look at issues of confidentiality when dealing with children and families. At the end of the chapter is a summary of the legislative backdrop to all our consultations involving children and young people. This is referenced for those who wish to find out more.

TERMS TO UNDERSTAND

1 Parental responsibility

The Children Act 1989 defines parental responsibility as 'all the rights, duties, powers, responsibilities and authority which by law a parent of a child has in relation to the child and his (the child's) property'.[1]

Parental responsibility is given to both the child's father and mother where they are married to each other at, or after, the child's conception. In the case of unmarried parents, the mother has parental responsibility. The father also has parental responsibility provided either his name is on the birth certificate (Adoption and Children Act 2002) or if he has acquired it via the courts or a parental responsibility agreement. A guardian who is appointed by the court or by a parent also acquires parental responsibility on taking up appointment.

2 'Gillick competence'

The Law Lords in 1985 gave a good summary of the concept of 'Gillick competence':

> [W]hether or not a child is capable of giving the necessary consent will depend on the child's maturity and understanding and the nature of the consent required. The child must be capable of making a reasonable assessment of the advantages and disadvantages of the treatment proposed, so the consent, if given, can be properly and fairly described as true consent.[2]

The term 'Gillick competence' has its origins in a case brought by a mother, Mrs Victoria Gillick, who went to court to ask that she have the right to know if her daughter (then under 16) requested contraceptive advice. She lost her case and her name has been given to the competence an under-16-year-old may have to consent, not only in the area of reproductive health, but now also more widely.

> As a matter of Law the parental right to determine whether or not their minor child below the age of sixteen will have medical treatment terminates if and when the child achieves sufficient understanding and intelligence to understand fully what is proposed.[2]
>
> Lord Scarman

Note: there are a number of things the child is required to understand. They must be able to:
➤ appreciate and consider the alternatives
➤ weigh up the pros and cons of each alternative
➤ express a clear and reasonably consistent view.

It is very important to give information at a level and in words that the child can understand before assuming that they cannot consent. Note also that this is not an all-or-nothing concept; a 14-year-old may be 'Gillick competent' to consent to one treatment (e.g. a course of antibiotics), but not to another (e.g. a heart transplant).

3 Fraser guidelines

One of the Law Lords in the Gillick case was Lord Fraser. He outlined some guidelines for the very specific situation of the giving of contraceptive advice and treatment to a girl under 16, which are still used by health professionals. A doctor could proceed to give advice and treatment provided he is satisfied in the following criteria:

1. that the girl (although under the age of 16 years of age) will understand his advice;
2. that he cannot persuade her to inform her parents or to allow him to inform the parents that she is seeking contraceptive advice;
3. that she is very likely to continue having sexual intercourse with or without contraceptive treatment;

4. that unless she receives contraceptive advice or treatment her physical or mental health or both are likely to suffer;
5. that her best interests require him to give her contraceptive advice, treatment or both without the parental consent.[2]

GILLICK AND FRASER COMPETENCE

There has been confusion regarding Gillick and Fraser competence. 'Gillick competence', while raised in the context of contraceptive advice, has for some time been used more widely and is now an accepted concept in all areas of medical treatment. The Fraser guidelines were derived specifically for contraceptive advice, although are now taken as pertaining to other areas of reproductive health including abortion. A story arose that Victoria Gillick objected to having her name attached to the competency. This led to the use of the term 'Fraser competence' instead. A recent *British Medical Journal* article would seem to suggest that this is not true and hence for this chapter I will use the original term.[3]

Informed Consent

The Department of Health has issued guidance on seeking consent when working with children.[4] To be able to give consent any person must be able to:
➤ comprehend and retain information material to the decision
➤ understand the consequences of having or not having the intervention in question
➤ use and weigh this information in the decision-making process
➤ make a voluntary uncoerced decision that remains reasonably consistent.

There is no specific age when a child becomes competent to consent to treatment. It depends both on the individual child and on the seriousness and complexity of the treatment being proposed. In younger children, the parent might be said to give informed permission with the assent of the child. Even a child who is not 'Gillick competent' may be helped to assent to treatment at the level of their understanding.[5]

In order to judge whether a child under 16 is sufficiently mature to give valid consent, it is useful to consider children's understanding of disease and to what extent they are able to make a free and independent decision without undue influence by parent or guardian. These issues were well covered by Kuther, in a review in 2003, who made the following points:
➤ young children cannot differentiate between symptoms and the causes of disease
➤ they may think disease is transmitted 'magically' or caused by misbehaviour
➤ as they get older they begin to understand causes of disease such as the connection between germs and infections
➤ how fast children's views of disease change and mature is very variable

➤ children who have had regular and frequent contact with doctors, perhaps as a result of chronic disease, can have more mature concepts
➤ it needs to be borne in mind that misunderstanding or confusion is not an inevitable consequence of cognitive immaturity
➤ a child may have the capacity to understand if the information is presented in an age-appropriate way.[6]

Younger children cannot readily consider hypothetical situations and will struggle to evaluate and select between several possible outcomes or alternatives. They also do not easily consider longer-term consequences. This ability appears gradually, usually around early adolescence.

There are a number of theories of the cognitive development of children, the most well known of which was developed by Jean Piaget. This is a complex field and a detailed review is beyond the scope of this chapter. There are a number of books exploring cognitive development, one of which, by Stephanie Thornton, is recommended in the Further Reading section at the end of this chapter.

It is also vital to consider whether a minor's consent is truly voluntary and that it is not constrained by others. Younger children usually consider parents and doctors as powerful and in authority, and will therefore comply with their wishes. These children are physically, emotionally and financially dependent on their parents and perhaps cannot be considered to make 'voluntary' decisions regarding consent. Conformity may peak at around 11 or 12 and decline thereafter. By adolescence, young people are more likely to question demands that seem unreasonable and are less susceptible to coercion.

The few studies comparing adolescent and adult decision-making show little difference in all these areas. By about 14 many adolescents perform comparably to older people in their ability to make rational choices.

CASE SCENARIO

A 14-year-old comes for a colonoscopy under general anaesthetic. At the time of getting the consent Mum readily agrees but the child in distress says he doesn't want it done. He can't express why not except to say over and over that he is frightened and doesn't want any of it. Mum says he is not normally like this, and can't believe there is any possibility the procedure might be cancelled, as she has given consent.
• Where do you stand legally as the anaesthetist or doctor doing the test?
• What would you do at this point?

Consent versus refusal

The Gillick ruling in law was concerned with who could give consent, rather than who could refuse. At present, consent can be from a person with parental responsibility, a 'Gillick competent' minor or the courts. This means that a 'Gillick competent' minor can give consent to a procedure, but if they refuse, the law allows for treatment to proceed, as long as a person with parental responsibility has consented on behalf of the minor. In other words, they can consent to, but not refuse treatment. In practice the refusal of a 'Gillick competent' minor is taken very seriously and only overturned if there are sufficient grounds.

Giving Consent

16–18 years

These young adults should be treated in exactly the same way as older adults. Many will rely to a greater or lesser extent on their parents' advice but they are presumed to be competent, unless they have a learning difficulty. Between the ages of 16 and 18, if they are felt not to have the capacity for informed consent, a person with parental responsibility can give consent on their behalf. After the age of 18 no one else can give consent and concepts of 'best interest' are used by clinicians.

12–16 years

From about age 12 a clinician will need to judge whether a child is 'Gillick competent'. As noted above, this becomes more likely from about age 14.

10–12 years

These children are much less likely to be 'Gillick competent' but this still must be considered by health professionals and consent obtained from them when this is appropriate.

Under 10 years

These children are usually presumed not to be 'Gillick competent' and consent is from someone with parental responsibility.

Refusing Consent

16–18 years

The refusal of these young people is treated in the same way as the refusal of an adult.

Under 16 years

If a 'Gillick competent' minor refuses but the person with parental responsibility consents, in theory you can go ahead. But in practice:
- it is hard to do anything to a non-consenting young person
- it is dangerous to discount their wishes and this may affect longer-term concordance
- parents find it very difficult and upsetting to be in this position.

With discussion and patience usually such conflicts can be resolved. If the procedure is for emergency or life-saving treatment, it can go ahead without permission. However, if time allows it is prudent to get the views of a legal advisor or of the courts. If it is an elective procedure it is best to postpone. Time invested at this stage to unpick the reasons for the refusal can pay dividends in the longer term and with patience usually results in agreement in the end. In the hospital setting involving a play specialist can be very helpful. Play specialists as part of their role prepare children for surgery and procedures by explaining what will happen. They are therefore well placed to take the time to listen to children and give information to allay fears, which in young people often revolve around anaesthetics and not waking up or waking in the middle of a procedure.

Bearing all these things in mind, we can summarise the situation with regard to giving consent at different ages as in the box 'Giving Consent'.[7]

Disagreements between parent, child and doctors regarding treatment

Situations can arise when parents (or 'Gillick competent' minors) disagree with health professionals about the best treatment or management of a medical condition. These situations are rare, but can cause a great deal of distress to all concerned and fall roughly into two categories:

1. Parent or competent child wants a treatment that the doctor feels is inappropriate.
2. Parent or competent child does not want a treatment that the doctor feels is necessary.

As above, time invested in thorough, careful discussion is very beneficial. The following need to be borne in mind in any discussion:

➤ the best interests of the child are paramount
➤ doctors can perform life-saving treatment even without permission from parents. All other treatment needs consent, as above
➤ the parents' or 'Gillick competent' child's wishes should be followed where possible
➤ a dying child's right to life does not require doctors to prolong treatment in all circumstances
➤ doctors have the right not to perform a treatment they feel to be futile
➤ sometimes the reasons given for wanting or not wanting a treatment can be legitimate and some degree of compromise can be reasonable.

Ultimately these situations will need to be decided by the courts, if agreement cannot be reached.

Brought for treatment by a person without parental responsibility

Parents (or others such as a foster-parent or social services, who may have parental responsibility) are not with their children 24 hours a day, and there are times when parents will devolve the responsibility to consent to treatment to others (e.g. grandparents or childminders) for certain interventions, such as emergency care and treatment of minor illness. Such consent does not need to be in writing and the health professional does not need to consult the parents, unless there is cause to believe the parents' views would differ significantly.

Where there is no specific agreement between parents and a third party in any given situation, the third party can give consent providing it can be justified as being in the best interests of the child. An example of this would be a teacher accompanying a child to the A&E department for urgent treatment required after an accident at school. If the treatment is not urgent then all efforts must be made to contact the parents to give consent, by telephone if necessary.

CONFIDENTIALITY

Confidentiality in consultations with 'Gillick competent' young people

In general, we must not use or disclose information that is given to us in confidence in a form that might identify patients without their consent and 'Gillick competent' children have the same right to this confidentiality as adults.[8]

We need to be sensitive to the young people who come to us unaccompanied. Fraser's guidelines regarding girls coming for contraceptive advice are obviously helpful here and require us to encourage them to disclose the treatment to their parents. If, however, a competent child under the age of 16 is insistent that their family should not be involved, their right to confidentiality must usually be respected. This remains true unless you can justify disclosure on the grounds that you have reasonable cause to suspect that the child is suffering, or is likely to suffer, significant harm.[9]

This is the crux of the matter. The doctor's primary duty is to act in the child's best interest – the child's needs are paramount. Disclosure of personal information without consent may be justified where failure to do so may expose the child or others to risk of serious harm.

CASE SCENARIO

A 15-year-old girl coming for contraceptive advice asks if a 10-year-old could get pregnant. After gentle discussion, she discloses possible sexual abuse, she thinks by an uncle who often visits the home, of her 10-year-old sister. She doesn't want you to tell anyone in the family or the police, because it would be obvious the information came from her.

- What would you do?
- What would you tell the young person?

Health professionals providing sexual health services must balance the child protection issues against the young person's right of confidentiality and their need for sexual healthcare – they may not seek the help they need if they feel confidentiality might be compromised. The Fraser guidelines above refer specifically to this situation, and guidelines for the practice of genitourinary medicine have been issued.[10] These suggest health professionals discuss the following:

➤ the emotional and physical implications of sexual activity, including the risks of pregnancy and sexually transmitted infections
➤ whether the relationship is mutually agreed and whether there may be coercion or abuse

➤ the benefits of informing their GP and the case for discussion with a parent or carer
➤ any refusal should be respected – in the case of abortion, where the young woman is competent to consent but cannot be persuaded to involve a parent, every effort should be made to help them find another adult to provide support, for example another family member or specialist youth worker
➤ any additional counselling or support needs.

Sexual activity in children under 13 is treated differently, as according to the Sexual Offences Act 2003 they are considered to be unable to consent to sexual activity. These should be taken on a case-by-case basis and strong consideration given to refer to Social Services.

Confidentiality in consultations with parents and younger children

The Human Rights Act applies to everyone, even younger children and their confidentiality should be respected as much as possible. The issue of confidentiality usually comes to the fore in cases where some kind of child abuse or the possibility of non-accidental injury exists. One example of this is when a child is thought to be in need. The legal definition is 'a child who, without services, is unlikely to achieve a reasonable standard of health or development, or whose health or development is likely to be significantly impaired', or, 'a child who is at risk of significant harm'.[3] In this circumstance you have a duty to inform Social Services. If you do decide that this is the correct course of action then you must let the parents know this is your intention.

CASE SCENARIO

A three-month-old presents for routine vaccinations. The nurse notices an obvious bump and small bruise on the forehead. Mum on questioning gets agitated and says he must have bumped it that morning when she was in the shower. The nurse is concerned about the minor head injury which has no satisfactory explanation, and his mother's behaviour when questioned about it.

- What should she do?
- What should she say to Mum?

There may be other occasions when sharing information with different professionals is deemed to be necessary – ideally this would be with a parent's consent, but if this is withheld, it may be necessary to share information anyway:

1. Early intervention and preventative services are needed when a family is identified as at-risk, or in need of extra support. This is now done using the Common Assessment Framework.
2. It is essential to the child's medical interests when it is clear that another health or other professional will need to be involved, or you need to take advice about a medical issue.
3. The information would help prevent, detect or prosecute a serious crime.

The exceptions to this are when you believe that it would increase the risk to the child or a sibling, that the person or other professionals caring for the child may come to harm, or that the child's verbal evidence may be interfered with by the parent. If handled sensitively most parents do understand the need to share information to detect the few cases where there is ongoing concern. This information sharing should be done according to the procedures of the Local Safeguarding Children Board. 'Often it is only when information from a number of sources has been shared and is then put together that it becomes clear that a child is at risk of or is suffering significant harm', as stated in paragraph 3.55.[11]

CASE SCENARIO

A mother brings her seven-month-old baby back to the health visitor to be weighed. Having previously been on the 50th centile the weight has gradually drifted down to the 2nd centile. The mother says he drinks good amounts of formula milk and has taken well to solids. She says the baby has no symptoms. The health visitor refers her to the GP at the time, who advises a blood test for anaemia. The mother refuses, saying, 'You're not hurting my baby', and gets up to leave.

- What would you do?

The following table is found on the 'Every Child Matters' website and is a good summary of the issues to consider in information sharing.[12]

Remember, wherever possible you should explain the problem, seek agreement and explain the reasons if you decide to act against a parent's or child's wishes. If in any doubt, seek advice from colleagues, professionals in other agencies or if necessary the court. Any action you take must be justifiable and carefully documented. Notes need to be legible, accurate and contemporaneous.

Seven golden rules for information sharing

1. Remember the Data Protection Act is not a barrier to sharing information.
2. Be open and honest with the person from the outset.
3. Seek advice where in doubt.
4. Share with consent where appropriate and where possible, respect the wishes of those who do not consent to share (unless there is sufficient need to override the lack of consent).
5. Always consider the safety and well-being of the person and others.
6. Ensure information is accurate and up to date, necessary, shared with the appropriate people, in a timely fashion and shared securely.
7. Record the reasons for the decision – whether it is to share or not.

Unintentional lapses in confidentiality

Finally, it is worth raising the issue of times when confidentiality is breached through external circumstances, or lack of thought. There are occasions when our conversations with families are in places where they can be easily overheard. This can lead to personal details and medical history being unintentionally shared with those around. There may be times when it is very difficult to avoid, but it is always worth checking if the child and family involved would wish the consultation be more private. On a ward this may mean moving to an office or treatment room, or asking others in the bay to move. Also phone conversations or informal discussions of a case can happen at a ward or reception desk, or in a canteen. We need to take care at these times that we discuss identifiable case details only in private.

LEGAL FRAMEWORK WHEN DEALING WITH CHILDREN

The following acts of parliament and guidelines provide the legal framework to our interactions with children and families.

1. The European Convention on Human Rights, which came into being in 1953, lists and defines universal human rights, which also apply to children.[13] These include among others:
   — The right to life, liberty, privacy and freedom of conscience and expression
   — The right to be protected from inhumane treatment or discrimination and protection from abuse in all its forms
   — The right for marriage and the family to be protected and the recognition that the welfare of any child is usually best served by supporting the family.
2. The Human Rights Act 1998 incorporated these rights into British law so that they must be adhered to in this country.[14] It became unlawful for a public authority to act in a way that contravenes any of these rights.
3. The Children Act 1989 introduced the concept of parental responsibility (rather than parental rights), and updated and coordinated the local authority's powers to safeguard children in need and provide services for children and families, in particular providing for 'looked-after' children.[3] One of the underlying principles is that the welfare of the child is paramount and any order made (such as care and supervision orders or child assessment or emergency protection orders) must be better for the child than not making the order.
4. The Children Act 2004 followed the Laming Report on the death of Victoria Climbie.[15] It aimed to provide integrated planning, commissioning and delivery of services, together with improved multidisciplinary working. It included the instigation of a 'children's commissioner' and the Local Safeguarding Children Boards. It also updated the inspection of children's services.
5. Some of our law is derived from legislation, the acts of parliament, but this is amplified and interpreted by the decisions of the courts. This part of law is referred to as 'common law'. The common-law duty of confidentiality requires there to be an 'overriding public interest' (as mentioned in the Freedom of Information Act)

or that there is a court order or other legal obligation in order for information given confidentially to be shared without permission.

6. The Data Protection Act 1998 gives the legal framework for the processing of personal data.[16] It states, for example, that such data should be accurate, not excessive, kept for no longer than necessary and kept securely.
7. Relevant national government guidelines include:
   — *Every Child Matters: change for children* gives wider aims for the welfare of children across the areas of health, social care, schools, etc.[17] It says that all children should: be healthy; stay safe; enjoy and achieve; make a positive contribution and achieve economic well-being.
   — *NSF (National Service Framework) for Children* (2004) gives more specific targets for the health service provision for children.[18] Its aims are to focus the care of children around the needs of children and families rather than the needs of organisations, to improve access and improve early intervention and to give children, young people and families increased information, power and choice.

CONCLUSION

Anyone who has dealings with children needs to have an understanding of these issues of consent and confidentiality, together with the legal framework that informs all our interactions. I have tried to summarise the main aspects, but it may be worth looking up the further reading or the summaries of some of the legislation if you would like to know more.

REFERENCES

1 Great Britain. Parliament. *Children Act 1989*. c.41.
2 Gillick vs. West Norfolk and Wisbech Area Health Authority and Department of Health and Social Security [1985] 3 WLR 830 [HL].
3 Wheeler R. Gillick or Fraser? A plea for consistency over competence in children. *Brit Med J*. 8 Apr 2006; **332**: 807.
4 Department of Health (DH). *Seeking Consent: working with children*. London: DH; November 2001.
5 Committee on Bioethics. Informed consent, parental permission, and assent in pediatric practice. *Pediatrics*. 1995; **95**(2): 314–17.
6 Kuther TL, Medical decision-making and minors: issues of consent and assent. *Adolescence*. 2003; **38**(150): 343–58.
7 Department of Health (DH). *Seeking Consent: working with children*. London: DH; Nov 2001.
8 General Medical Council (GMC). *Good Practice Guide*. London: GMC; May 2001.
9 Royal College of Paediatrics and Child Health (RCPCH). *Responsibilities of Doctors in Child Protection Cases with Regard to Confidentiality*. London: RCPCH; Feb 2004.
10 Department of Health (DH). *GUM Guidelines Best Practice Guidance for Doctors and Other*

Health Professionals on the Provision of Advice and Treatment to Young People Under 16 on Contraception, Sexual and Reproductive Health. London: DH; 2004.

11 Department of Health (DH). *Working Together to Safeguard Children: a guide to inter-agency working to safeguard and promote the welfare of children.* London: DH *et al.*; 1999.

12 Department for Education and Skills (DfES). *Every Child Matters.* London: The Stationery Office; 2003.

13 Convention for the Protection of Human Rights and Fundamental Freedoms, 4 Nov 1950. 213 U.N.T.S 222, C.E.T.S. 5.

14 Great Britain. Parliament. *Human Rights Act.* 1998. c.42.

15 Great Britain. Parliament. *Children Act.* 2004. c.31.

16 Great Britain. Parliament. *Data Protection Act.* 1998. c.29.

17 Department for Education and Skills (DfES). *Every Child Matters.* London: The Stationery Office; 2003.

18 Department of Health (DH). *The National Service Framework for Children, Young People and Maternity Services.* London: DH; 2004.

FURTHER READING

1 British Medical Association. *Consent, Rights and Choices in Health Care for Children and Young People.* London: BMJ Books; Dec 2000 (ISBN 0 7279 1228 3).

2 Royal College of Paediatrics and Child Health (RCPCH). *Responsibilities of Doctors in Child Protection Cases with Regard to Confidentiality.* London: RCPCH; Feb 2004.

3 Donovan C, Suckling HC. *Difficult Consultations with Adolescents.* Oxford: Radcliffe Medical Press; 2004.

4 Royal College of General Practitioners and Brook. *Confidentiality and Young People: improving teenagers' uptake of sexual and other health services. A toolkit for general practice, primary care groups and trusts.* London: Department of Health; 2000.

5 Thornton S. *Growing minds: an introduction to children's cognitive development.* New York: Palgrave MacMillan; 2003.

CHAPTER 9

Safeguarding children: heeding the messages

Adrian Brooke and Elizabeth Anderson

INTRODUCTION

Protecting children who are being harmed by adults is one of the greatest challenges facing professionals who work with children. Detecting that abuse is happening requires expertise in communication and judgement in deciding how to respond. The skills of listening to children, to hear their voices, are necessary to make the initial diagnosis. Effective action demands good verbal and written communication with colleagues particularly, as there are many obstacles to the exchange of high-quality information.

As well as the traditional barriers of territorialism between disciplines and time pressure from overwork there are a number of new issues. There has been major change in the way services are structured with the creation of Sure Start programmes and children centres. These have disrupted established patterns of work between different health professionals. Other changes such as the European Working Time Directive and a substantial increase in the number of general practitioners, most of who only work part-time, limit the opportunities for individuals to talk to each other. A more rapid turnover of staff in both health and social care professions means that people stay for shorter periods of time in one area with fewer opportunities to 'learn the patch' and, in the case of health visiting, there has been a 13.5% drop in the workforce in the past four years.[1,2] This further reduces consistency and continuity.

This chapter describes the main forms of child abuse and highlights that in this field there is often conflict between the needs of children and the wishes of the adults who are their carers. It describes the principles of early identification and effective assessment of cases where abuse is suspected, illustrated by case vignettes. It finishes by describing the centrality of good interprofessional working practice in protecting abused children.

FORMS OF ABUSE

The various forms of abuse encountered in paediatric practice are neglect, physical, emotional and sexual abuse and fabricated or induced illness. Neglect may be suspected where one sees an abandoned child, or one with unsuitable clothing. Children may come with animal bites, or may be dirty, have poor hygiene (including oral hygiene and dental caries), fail to thrive, or present with faltering growth. Such children may not attend for immunisation, health promotion or scheduled health reviews or there may be problems with medication concordance. It should be suspected when home conditions are inadequate for the needs of the child (including lack of food, appropriate safety measures or toys appropriate for the child's developmental age) or where there is concern about lack of supervision.

Physical abuse encompasses cuts, abrasions and lacerations, bites and teeth marks, burns, scalds, bruises and petechiae, fractures and head injuries. Additional forms of physical abuse include thermal injuries, ligature marks and strangulation, injuries to the mouth or eyes and injuries to the spine, thorax or abdomen. Scarring may represent old injuries that have escaped previous attention.

Emotional abuse is where the child may encounter persistent belittling or unwarranted criticism. Behaviour may not be appropriate for the child's age (including inappropriate sexual behaviour) or there may be excessive aggression or passivity. Some children may rock or have other stereotyped movements while others may self-harm. Children may have toileting problems including enuresis, encopresis and smearing of faeces.

Sexual abuse may be suspected when sexualised behaviours are seen that are inappropriate for the age of the child, or where there are complaints of dysuria, or discharge from the genitalia or anus. There may be problems with constipation or soiling, abdominal pain, pregnancy and sexually transmitted diseases. There may be evidence of physical abuse in the ano-genital region, breasts or mouth.

In fabricated or induced illness the child is presented to doctors with a history suggesting a significant illness, but objective assessment (history from other carers, examination, assessment and investigation) does not tally with the story told by the parent. Some aspects of this form of abuse overlap with areas covered within emotional abuse.

In all the examples cited (and the list is not exhaustive), the presence of one or more of these features does not necessarily indicate definite abuse; rather, it should prompt the professional to consider the possibility carefully and then to judge whether further discussion with other professionals is indicated.

CONFLICTING NEEDS

In most areas of professional practice it is essential to communicate effectively with children and their parents to reach a shared understanding of the child's problem and what can be done to address it.[3] Generally the needs of both the child and parent are closely aligned. A unique characteristic of practice in safeguarding children is that the child's predicament may be a direct result of conflict between the needs of the child and the attitudes or wishes of the parent, often leading to physical and emotional damage to the child. The results range from insidious, low-level but long-lasting damage to a child's self-esteem through emotional abuse to physical assault causing serious injury or death. This resolution of the tension between the needs of the child and those of the parents is enshrined in law in the Children Act 1989 which states that the 'needs of the child are paramount'. This guiding principle includes all other potential carers such as foster carers, grandparents and adoptive parents.

Despite this simple maxim children continue to come to harm at the hands of their parents, while in full view of health and social-care professionals because those involved with the family are unable to separate the needs of the adults from those of the child. For example, in the case of Baby Peter, a 17-month-old boy was murdered despite being subject to a child protection plan and being seen by professionals from both health and social care on no fewer than 60 occasions. Lord Laming articulated the requirement for professionals to appreciate this restriction on the rights of parents in his report into the death of Victoria Climbié when he coined the phrase 'respectful uncertainty'.[4]

> The concept of respectful uncertainty should lie at the heart of the relationship between the social worker and the family. It does not require social workers constantly to interrogate their clients but it does involve the critical evaluation of information that they are given. People who abuse their children are unlikely to inform social workers of the fact. For this reason at least social workers must keep an open mind. (p. 205)[4]

Although Lord Laming is referring to social workers, the notion of 'respectful uncertainty' is necessary for all professionals dealing with abused children. A full understanding of the implications of this concept must be central to the approach taken when safeguarding children; it should inform the communication strategy used with both the child and the parents.

IDENTIFICATION AND ASSESSMENT

CASE VIGNETTE 1

Bobby attends school in summer clothing during a cold winter term. The teacher discusses her concerns with the school nurse who sees the child with her mother and observes that the child presents in dirty clothes, with lank hair infested with head lice, in a state of poor hygiene. After a discussion with the child's mother (who it transpires has her own mental health issues) a referral is made to social care to investigate the possibility that she is at risk of neglect.

Health professionals who deal with children will come across those being harmed by their parents in a variety of ways and in different settings. The spectrum can range from a health visitor becoming concerned at a baby failing to gain weight in a community clinic, through to an intensive care nurse noticing apparent parental indifference to a child's life-threatening injuries and a primary school teacher who notices a change in a child's emotional state. The ability to recognise the possibility of child abuse is as important as the skill to assess and manage suspected cases.

Once the possibility of abuse is considered, it is mandatory to discuss these concerns with more experienced colleagues – all public services that work with children, from hospital and primary care trusts to nurseries and schools, have named professionals with specific responsibility for safeguarding children and young people within the organisation. When a school nurse or health visitor sees a child they are doing so on behalf of their employing health organisation so they can relate any concerns where necessary to senior members of their team or to the organisation's named professional. The content and outcome of these discussions should be clearly recorded. Children are put at greater risk when these conclusions are not effectively communicated and shared with other professionals who work with the child or young person to alert them and identify any further episodes which might heighten the level of concern. For example, if a nursing professional reports a concern about a suspicious bruise on a child they should record the concern and the conversation regarding the concern with their senior colleague, whose identity, role and advice should also be noted. The record of the concern should form the factual basis for referral to the appropriate investigating agency (often social care) and the outcome of the discussion with these colleagues should also be recorded. Then all those who work with the child should be asked to pool their knowledge of the current whole picture relating to the child.

CASE VIGNETTE 2

Alice is four. The school nurse has been asked to look at a faint, diffuse bruise on her face by the Early Years teacher. When asked how she got the bruise she looks down at her feet and says, 'I fell down'. Despite encouragement she cannot give any more details. When Mum comes to collect her, the nurse asks, 'What happened to Alice?' and she replies, 'Oh, she ran into the door this morning'. The discrepancy between the two accounts and the fact the bruise does not have the right shape means that further investigation is needed.

During the assessment of children suspected of being abused the aims of the consultation are to obtain a history of relevant events from the parent and, wherever possible, the child. The history should be obtained independently from both and allow the child to describe any alleged abuse or injuries in a fully supported and unpressured environment, away from possible coercion at the hands of the parents and/or the alleged perpetrator. However, it is also important to observe the interaction between parent and child as inferences can be drawn from this important dynamic. Once a clear understanding of how the child has come to present has been gained, an examination should be carried out to assess any injury. For example, if a child has bruises the parent should explain the cause of bruising and then a history is obtained from the child.

A key point in the assessment is the reconciliation of the history with any findings on examination to see if one explains the other. Accurate recording of the history is vital and accounts of how injuries were sustained should be documented, identifying who has said what, and when. Conflicting stories of how an injury was sustained from several carers or a changing story are often encountered in cases of physical abuse. Often the injuries found on examination do not tally with the history offered. Importantly the child may give a different explanation from the parents. When such injuries are not consistent with the parental history the examining professional should try to ascribe a plausible mechanism for any injuries seen and decide whether the presentation is likely to be indicative of abuse or not.

Health and social care professionals often forget that school teachers spend more time with children from age four onwards than any other professional. They are therefore very well placed to detect the signs that a child may be experiencing abuse (see Box 9.1).

BOX 9.1 Changes of behaviour communicating stress as noticed by both primary and secondary school teachers

- Poor attendance or consistent late arrival.
- Changes in mood from quiet and withdrawn, or the opposite, angry and aggressive. Poor personal hygiene.
- A child who becomes isolated in the year group or on the fringe in the playground.
- Drop in standard of work.
- Weight changes which are significant, either gain or loss.
- A child who begins to hang back at the end of the lesson and wants to talk or is seeking protection by being near to the teacher.
- Signs of self-harm, picking spots, scabs on skin.
- A complete change in appearance, e.g. dyed hair, intense make-up, change of dress.
- Stunted psychological or physical growth.
- Sudden speech impediment.
- Fantasy stories, e.g. creates a make-believe brother, sister and imaginary friends.
- Hearing voices.
- Bringing a security object from home.
- Cues with anger management, break down of respect to adults and peer group..
- Running away and more serious incidents like overdoses.

The ability to detect the possibility of abuse is an essential attribute of all professionals working with children and young people. A fundamental requirement for success is to have expertise in communication skills. This involves detecting subtle nuances in what children say and do and knowing how to respond to these in such a way that the child concerned trusts the adult to be protecting them.

CASE VIGNETTE 3

Marcus is six and with Anna in the Wendy house. The play worker overhears him asking her to take off her knickers so he can see her 'minny'. She takes him to a quiet room and gently asks him about the game he was playing. He says it is a game that Vicky plays with him when she is babysitting. Later investigation reveals that Vicky is 13 and was sexually abused by her uncle for several years.

It is important to realise that the investigation of possible child abuse is regulated by civil law and therefore the burden of probability required to 'prove' abuse is lower than under criminal law. While in criminal cases abuse should be likely 'beyond reasonable doubt', in civil cases proceedings to safeguard the child can occur if abuse is 'more likely than not'. Thus, the investigating professional does not need to possess absolute certainty that the injury is non-accidental; rather, they must be able to demonstrate that the injury or presentation is more likely due to abuse than not.

Health professionals may be involved at the outset by becoming suspicious of abuse (and thereby detecting it) through to the comprehensive assessment and forensic examination of children referred following detection of abuse. The need to keep clear records that can be used in courts of law as evidence is vital and hence an ability to communicate effectively with all parties (social worker, health professional, teacher, relatives, parent and child) is extremely important.

It is therefore evident that the faithful recording of the child's account of the events leading up to the presentation is of central importance. Every effort should be made to speak to the child on their own, as it is widely acknowledged that children and young people are participants in their own right. This requirement for the separate ascertainment of the history and wishes from the child contrasts starkly with the approach elsewhere in paediatric practice.

It must be realised that although some health professionals both recognise and assess cases of child abuse, in most instances those recognising the possibility of abuse are different from those who are then asked to make specific assessments and carry out the multi-agency work required to safeguard the child or young person.

For professions involved in the assessment of suspected cases of child abuse, additional sensitivities pertain. For example, in alleged cases of child sexual abuse where a forensic examination of the anus and genitals is required, the examiner needs to be mindful that the procedure should be carried out as sensitively and patiently as possible to avoid further unnecessary trauma to the victim. It is for this reason that in many centres child sexual abuse investigations are carried out jointly by a specially trained paediatrician and a forensic medical examiner so that an appropriate examination and collection of forensic samples can be done just once to avoid the repeated trauma of several intimate examinations.

During Lord Laming's recent report into the progress of child protection services in England, he pointedly noted that it was not further legislation that was required to protect children. Effective protection of children will come from the vigilance and prompt action of the many professionals they meet.[5]

Children in the care of the local authority

This group of children consists of those where the local authority assumes the role of parent and thereby becomes the legal guardian of the child. The accommodation of these children within the birth family is either wholly or partly impossible and includes those subject to child abuse and neglect. Such children form a vulnerable population and have demonstrably poorer outcomes in terms of physical, emotional and mental health, educational achievement, employment as young adults and social inclusion. The babies, children and young people may be accommodated with birth relatives (other than those who have abused them), fostered, placed in children's homes or occasionally secure accommodation. Their experiences, predicament and circumstances often mean that communication with this vulnerable group is difficult and special sensitivities are required in the approach to offering them appropriate access to healthcare.

Often, the staff who have recognised or assessed cases of abuse are then called upon to work with families who are subject to child protection plans. In this situation, there are additional challenges to those that exist in maintaining a relationship between the family and health services, as the very fact that recognition of abuse has occurred may have fractured what was a carefully nurtured relationship between the two parties. While the professionals may wish to rebuild this trust, they also need to be mindful of both the parents' views and the child's views about progress made against any plans within the child protection framework and also in the event of further episodes of harm or abuse.

Against this complex cocktail of legal requirement and emotional need, the professionals may forget to maintain an adequate degree of 'respectful uncertainty' when working with the family. Framing the approach to the family with this need will ensure that the needs of the child are not lost in attempting to support the family during the process of ongoing child protection and rehabilitation.

INTERPROFESSIONAL COMMUNICATION

High-quality team working is fundamental to safeguard children. Virtually all reviews of fatal child abuse cases highlight poor team working, particularly the quality of communication between practitioners.[6] The subsequent government enquiries have considered that solutions to these problems might arise through the redesign of health services to emphasise collaboration across all relevant statutory services, including social care and schools.[7,8] However, many argue that these errors relate to poor interprofessional working which cannot be solved through policy change.[9] Much of this evidence indicates that the following are important reasons for defective communication:[9-11]

➤ lack of clarity, accuracy and consistency of data exchanged
➤ professionals whose frame of thinking about the case varies significantly

➤ mistrust and lack of respect between professions
➤ poor understanding of confidentiality, consent and referral processes
➤ territorialism
➤ status and power
➤ competition for resources and professional and organisational priorities.

The psychosocial aspects of poor interprofessional communication listed above bear some remarkable similarities with our professional problems in developing highly skilled approaches to communicating with children and young people. In particular, the effective transfer of information between two professionals depends upon what is said being understood by the person hearing it. A paediatrician reflected at the Lord Laming inquiry, 'I cannot account for the way people interpreted what I said. It was not the way I would have liked it to have been interpreted' (p. 9).[4]

This stage of the inquiry addressed the inadequate clarity of clinical messages passed between medical colleagues and then on to social services. Here the consultant paediatrician was convinced that Victoria had scabies but failed to speak with her colleague who earlier in the day had considered the possibility of non-accidental injury. The consultant asked a registrar to write up the notes, which read, 'no child protection' issues, but actually meant no physical abuse issues. The subsequent discharge letter to social services lacked clarity so that police protection was withdrawn and no full investigation took place.

The emotional impact of communicated messages can make them hard to hear and heavily depends upon the intellectual ability and emotional intelligence of the professional to discern the difference between important and incidental aspects of the message. Timing and context affect emotional impact so that giving a vital message at the end of the day or during a busy episode, with little time for reflection, should be avoided. This was indeed the case on several occasions with Victoria Climbié when staff going off duty failed to speak to those left in charge. Morrison expressed this type of emotional distraction in communication as follows: 'working together means contact between differing emotional realities, different systems of meaning and different types of bias' (p. 130).[12]

Communication with children and their families mostly relates to one moment in time associated with the reason for the dialogue, for example a doctor taking a history or a nurse admitting a patient. At different moments between and across professions messages become lost. There is often no single coherent body of knowledge relating to the exchange of information between the child and family and the interprofessional team. In this way no meaning is given to all the information gathered and no action taken. While Victoria was an in-patient different members of the nursing and medical teams simply failed to speak to one another.

> The reciprocal interplay between communication and assessment mindsets runs vividly and uncomfortably through the Victoria Climbié case. On many occasions, misunderstandings between professionals about the nature of her injuries framed how the case was viewed and the nature of the assessments that were needed.[4] (p. 428)

There were numerous failures to ensure that things they thought would happen did happen. Victoria's case clearly demonstrates the need for doctors and nurses to document information, action and referrals consistently and unambiguously, to share that information and to ensure subsequently that what has been agreed is carried through.[4] (p. 283)

A further danger to effective communication is that each discipline can form a different relationship with different members of the family, while seeking to identify the truth for the child. These differing perceptions and the interplay of these exchanges can confuse the truth: 'family members impart selected information to various professionals, each of whom believes that they understand the family well, not realising that they are only seeing a fragment of the picture' (p. 93).[5]

Lord Laming made 108 recommendations to improve child protection, mostly around changes in the way services are structured and organised and emphasising the need for effective joined-up thinking and working within and across disciplines. These have led to new legislation and the establishment of local Children's Trusts (interprofessional services for delivering care to children and young people), with an emphasis on how confidential information is shared. Within each area the Children's Trusts are accountable to the Local Safeguarding Children's Board (LSCB) to account for how they monitor and ensure safeguarding processes within their trust. The LSCB is a high-level strategic group of professionals across health, social care, policing and education who translate government policy locally into strategic safeguarding plans. They monitor the quality of services from performance data returned by the Children's Trusts. After the second Lord Laming report following the death of Baby Peter these processes are being refined into new 'Working Together' policies. The whole review process will further improve services to children and families and aims to focus on the child. Consider the case in Box 9.2, and the pathway of professional responsibilities.

BOX 9.2 Interprofessional communication

An inner-city, single-parent mother with five children was in contact with the family GP, health visitor, youth worker and primary school teachers. The eldest child, at 15 years of age, was permanently excluded from school while the younger children (aged four, six and eight years) appeared at first to be well cared for. The referral for social work involvement followed discussion between the health visitor and GP. There had been a change in the younger children emotionally and physically with increased visits to the GP by the mother. At the child protection conference, the GP shared data on recent missed health screening appointments for the mother and young children, physical development of the children and maternal health factors of obesity, smoking and concern about recent excessive alcohol intake resulting in accident and emergency admissions. In addition, the social worker found that a previous male partner had returned to the family home and fuelled tensions between the older teenage child, mother and young siblings. There were concerns for the safety of the younger children in the house. These concerns mirrored the teacher's records of late arrival at school and observed emotional distress in the young children. The health visitor's records affirmed those of both the social worker and teacher concerning home tension and increase in her observation of stress within the home and family. The pooled assessments enabled sensible shared decisions resulting in the teenager being temporarily given residential placement while family dynamics were collectively assessed.

THE PATHWAY OF CHILD PROTECTION
Step 1

In this case the health visitor came to discuss the family with the GP. This highlights good practice enabling clear accurate sharing of professional records between professionals in contact with the child and family because they have identified that there is a possible child protection issue.

Process
Each professional has a duty under the children's acts of 1989 and 2004 to cooperate and share information for the best outcomes of the child, which is endorsed by each profession's Royal College.

Problems
New children centres have removed many health visitors from GP premises and opportunities for face-to-face meetings are reduced and require more effort to establish and maintain.

Step 2

The sharing of information results in a consensus that there is sufficient concern to alert social services. A joint assessment in writing and by telephone is made to social services. Both the GP and health visitor separately document the meeting in their professional record.

Process
Each profession is accountable for keeping contemporaneous accounts of meetings involving child protection concerns.

Problems
There remain separate profession-specific records and no shared documents.

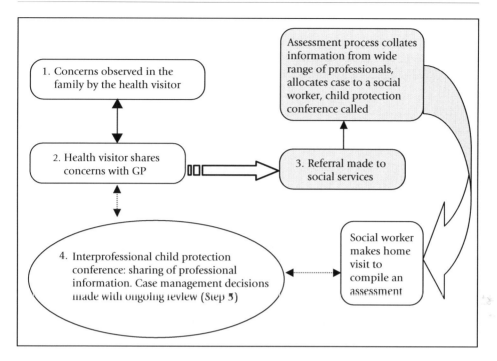

FIGURE 9.1 Monitoring and supporting the family

Step 3

A social work assessment of the situation includes a home visit and the gathering of information from all those who know the child and family. In this case the local youth workers and school teachers. This information is shared with senior colleagues and a child protection conference is called.

Process

Social work must fulfil its obligations to investigate any referral. In this case the social worker does this and speaks to all the professionals involved and calls a child protection conference

Problems

Each profession must share exactly how they view the situation. In many cases the family may be viewed differently by different professions according to how they work with them and know them. Each professional should prepare their own report ahead of the case conference and not engage with or collude with others concerning their perceptions.

Step 4

All come together to present their own profession-specific knowledge concerning the children in the family. Each professional writes a document to be shared which can be substantiated from their own professional records. A joint decision is agreed and a way forward with clear action plans is documented.

Step 5

All work to the agreed action plan which will be cyclically reviewed together.

Process

The case conference should bring together a range of professionals who know the family and who bring a healthy scepticism to the meeting. The pooling of information is required so that the range of perspectives can be explored.

Problems

Following the death of Baby Peter, Lord Laming stated that professions had often not kept an open mind and were guilty of colluding with one another. The child protection conference needs to ensure full attendance of all professions. However, many continue to state that the timing of these meetings prevents their attendance, for example GPs and teachers.

Finally, although interprofessional communication remains paramount, in many situations it has been the system within which safeguarding of children and young people takes place that have led to errors. By system we mean the features of professional tasks, tools and their working environment. The system also encompasses how professionals are expected to act and, if unpacked, can offer insights into the strengths and weaknesses of factors which bind working lives and become translated into what is not done rather than what should be done within a thinking, reflective system. The system also includes how individual actions are communicated and how multi-agency working takes place. It has been proposed that using a multi-agency systems approach for case reviews might promote learning together to safeguard children.[13]

CONCLUSIONS

The safeguarding of children is by its very nature a contentious area of practice for health and social care professionals. The needs of the child must remain uppermost in the minds of the professional workers and all those involved must accept their duty in the recognition and management of child abuse investigations. Maintaining a sensitive approach that allows the views of the child to be heard must be balanced with the predicament of the parents, while ensuring the need for objectivity.

In order to prevent further injuries and even death to children, better training and preparation for communication is required, with an emphasis on the experience of the child in both pre- and post-qualified health and social care education.[14,15] The second report by Lord Laming following the inquiry into the death of Baby Peter states:

> [S]taff often do not have the time needed to maintain effective contact with children, young people and their families in order to achieve positive outcomes. In these circumstances professionals can find it very difficult to take the time to assess the family environment through the eyes of a child or young person. The failure to see the situation from their perspective and talk to them was highlighted in Ofsted's first annual report of Serious Case Reviews . . . as far as possible they (staff) must put themselves in the place of the child or young person and consider first and foremost how the situation must feel to them. (p. 22)[5]

The institutional response necessary to overcome these difficulties is to improve pre- and post-qualification training using an interprofessional approach. This is a necessary prerequisite step to allow procedural and managerial changes to operate to prevent future system failures that result in preventable injury and death of children.

Learning to communicate in challenging situations requires a range of techniques and skills. The most effective of these require one-to-one or small-group practical sessions. Analysis of video-recorded interactions in the workplace, the use of simulated patients and facilitated role play are techniques that have a powerful effect on learners. They heighten awareness of skill deficiencies and provide opportunity for practice following specific feedback. Sadly, too often each discipline works in isolation and the opportunity to exchange these skills in interprofessional learning settings is lost. There remains little alignment on content and little vision as to how each professional group might support each other to enhance communication with children and young people. In essence, as Reder and Duncan state:

> In the long run, interagency communication would improve if all professionals concerned acquired a 'communication mindset' as part of their core skills. It is, admittedly, a well-rehearsed recommendation that training is key to such improvements: but it is true. Practitioners need to be able to consider their work in context and the ethos that 'I am part of a system' must be ingrained in professionals' minds so that it becomes automatic thinking. In addition, training time needs to be devoted to the interprofessional skills of communicating, such as monitoring what and how one conveys information, how one listens to another professional and how other people's messages are interpreted. Such training would need to occur at both prequalifying and post qualifying levels and include the different professions training together so that they could reflect on prejudgements that they held about each other and how these intrude into interagency coordination.[9]

The ability to improve communication with children and young people and then ensure effective interprofessional communication needs to be conducted within systems which enable rather than constrain professional working lives.

REFERENCES

1 Cowley S. Say 'health visiting'. *Pract*. 2010; **83**(1): 30–1.
2 Cowley S, Dowling S, Caan W. Too little for early interventions? Examining the policy–practice gap in English health visiting services and organisation. *Prim Health Care Res Dev*, 2009; **10**(2): 130–42.
3 McNeish D, Newman T. Involving children and young people in decision-making. In: McNeish D, Newman T, Roberts H (editors). *What Works for Children?* Buckingham Open University Press; 2002. pp. 187–206.
4 Laming. *The Victoria Climbié Inquiry Report of an Inquiry by Lord Laming*. Secretary of State for Health and Secretary for the Home Department. CM5730. London: The Stationery Office; 2003.
5 Laming. *The Protection of Children in England: a progress report*. HC330. London: The Stationery Office; 2009.
6 Parton N. From Maria Colwell to Victoria Climbié: reflections on public inquiries into child abuse a generation apart. *Child Abuse Rev*. 2004; **13**: 80–94.
7 Department for Education and Skills (DfES). *Common Core of Skills and Knowledge for the Children's Workforce*. Nottingham: DfES; 2005.
8 Department for Education and Skills. *Every Child Matters*. London: The Stationery Office; 2003.
9 Reder P, Duncan S. Understanding communication in child protection. *Child Abuse Rev*. 2003; **12**: 82–100.
10 Reder P, Maitra B. Barriers to working together. *Clin Child Psychol Psychiatr*. 2000; **5**: 453–5.
11 Richardson S, Asthana S. Inter-agency information sharing in health and social care services: the role of professional culture. *Brit J Soc Work*. 2006; **36**: 657–9.
12 Morrison T. Partnership and collaboration: rhetoric and reality. *Child Abuse Negl*. 1996; **20**: 127–40.
13 Fish S, Munro E, Bairstow S. Learning together to safeguard children: developing a multi-agency systems approach for case reviews. London: Social Care institute for Excellence (SCIE); 2008.
14 Priest H, Sawyer A, Roberts P, *et al*. A survey of interprofessional education in communication skills in healthcare programmes in the UK. *J Interprof Care*. 2005; **19**(3): 236–50.
15 Taylor I, Whiting R, Sharland E. *Integrated Children's Services in Higher Education Project: knowledge review*. Southampton: Higher Education Subject Centre for Social Policy and Social Work; 2008.

CHAPTER 10

Communication challenges: overcoming disability

Heather Benjamin and Dorothy MacKinlay

INTRODUCTION

This chapter focuses on health professionals' consultations with children and young people with learning difficulties. There is an overview of helpful techniques for health professionals consulting with children and young people with special needs. It explores in depth the authors' work with children and young people with severe learning difficulties and the techniques used to communicate with them. It further examines the different dynamics of consulting with children and young people as patients and the roles of parents, carers and siblings.

United Nations Convention on the Rights of the Child (1989)

Article 12
States Parties shall assure to the child who is capable of forming his or her own views the right to express those views freely in all matters affecting the child, the views of the child being given due weight in accordance with the age and maturity of the child.

Article 13
The child shall have the right to freedom of expression; this right shall include freedom to seek, receive and impart information and ideas of all kinds, regardless of frontiers, either orally, in writing or in print, in the form of art, or through any other media of the child's choice.

The rights of all children and young people are enshrined in the United Nations Convention on the Rights of the Child.[1] In the UK, as far back as 1976, the Court

Report advocated the need for every child to achieve their potential and for services for children with special needs to be coordinated around the child.[2] In 2005, an amendment to the Disability Discrimination Act made it unlawful for any organisation or service provider to treat disabled people less favourably than other people because of their disability.[3] It also requires them to make reasonable adjustments to make their services accessible to disabled people. The recent transformation programme for disabled children's services, Aiming High for Disabled Children, also emphasised the need for services to be built around the child.[4] It was jointly developed by the Department of Education, Schools and Families and the Department of Health and published in 2007.

Although policy-makers want disabled children and young people to be a priority both nationally and locally, it is often difficult for health professionals to put this agenda into practice, as many do not receive training in communication with people with special needs.[4] It is not always easy to find readily accessible resources (such as a guide to sign systems like Makaton) to facilitate this process. These practical barriers can also be accompanied by emotional barriers. The able-bodied can have many misconceptions about those with special needs, which can be challenged when people with special needs are given the opportunity to express themselves. The Study of Participation of Children with Cerebral Palsy Living in Europe (SPARCLE) is a nine-centre European epidemiological research study examining the relationship of participation and quality of life to impairment and environment (physical, social and attitudinal) in 8–12-year-old children with cerebral palsy.[5] When these young people with cerebral palsy were given the opportunity to comment on their quality of life using an appropriate measure, the results showed that they assessed this differently to their parents. Typically, the children assessed their own quality of life as higher than their parents did.

This reinforces the need not to make assumptions but to engage in communication with young people in such a way that their voices can be heard. This chapter provides guidance on how to create an opportunity for this to happen. It is founded on a psychoeducational approach and draws on the combined experience of a teacher of children with special needs and a clinical psychologist. Together we have worked therapeutically with children with complex needs who demonstrate behavioural challenges.

PREPARING FOR THE CONSULTATION

Ideally, health professionals should have prior knowledge of a child or young person's needs in order to prepare both themselves and the environment before the consultation starts. Good preparation can avoid problems which could interfere with a successful consultation. It is important to remember that young people with special needs often have more than one difficulty. The health professional should therefore take into account any co-morbidity issues. A young person with cerebral palsy may be in a wheelchair and if their speech is affected, they may also need a communication aid in order to participate fully in the consultation. The list below outlines some of the features that health professionals might like to consider prior to the consultation.

➤ Access and space: wheelchair access may be required and the room should be big enough to make seating arrangements comfortable and wheelchair manoeuvres as easy as possible. Toilet facilities should be easily accessible.

➤ Lighting: this may be important especially for people with visual difficulties. The opportunity to close curtains may also be helpful for those where visual glare or distraction is an issue.

➤ Noise: a quiet environment is obviously important for the hearing impaired but may also be relevant for those who are easily distracted.

➤ Seating arrangement: face-to-face is often best but would be less appropriate for someone who only has peripheral vision, for example. Choice may be important as with young people with autistic spectrum disorder (ASD).

➤ Communication aids: it is useful to establish beforehand what communication aids are required and ensure that these can be used during the consultation.

Issues for particular patient groups

Children and young people can demonstrate a range of different special needs and learning disabilities and it would be unusual for health professionals working in a generic setting to have sufficiently wide experience in dealing with all possibilities. Consequently, it is advisable to ask the young person or the person accompanying the child to inform you about the best way to achieve successful communication in the session. This is preferable to making assumptions that may impede the process or cause upset. It can also be very useful to establish if the child or young person uses hearing aids, glasses or communication aids. If these are used regularly they should have been brought to the consultation. If not, then this is also a relevant topic for discussion.

Deaf and hearing impaired

Hearing can be impaired to various degrees, ranging from mild to severe, and can be present from birth or acquired subsequently. The nature of hearing impairment will determine the type of communication aid required. Hearing aids may be used but some people will use lip-reading and/or sign language. Children and young people with profound hearing loss from birth will have more difficulty in acquiring speech. Even if speech is not present, the child or young person may be able to understand and use visual symbols or sign systems. Health professionals might like to consider the following guidance when consulting with hearing impaired persons.

➤ Early discussion to explore what is appropriate for each individual is important as well as to establish what term they prefer to use to describe their condition.

➤ A quiet environment with few distractions or extraneous noises. With hearing aids all sounds are amplified and appropriate sound selection may be difficult.

➤ Seating: opposite may be best (face-to-face and eye level) especially for lip-reading and signing. Avoid unnecessary movement and visual redundancy.

➤ Consider what communication aids are necessary? Does the person use hearing aids, lip-reading or signing?

➤ If the child or young person does not have speech, do they make use of visual referencing or a voice output communication aid (VOCA)?

Visually impaired

Vision can be impaired in a variety of ways and to various degrees. However, most children and young people considered visually impaired have some useable vision. Those termed blind often can tell the difference between light and dark. The nature of some young people's visual difficulties may mean that they use their peripheral vision and thus may need to turn their head to view things better. Glasses may have been prescribed.

A visual impairment can affect how a child learns. Where eye contact is reduced or not present, this represents an additional challenge. Without eye contact, it is hard to tell if a child or young person is paying attention. Children and young people with visual impairments may also miss visual cues, such as a frown, raised eyebrows, or smiles or other facial or body language which is used to communicate with others. Waving, pointing and nodding can also create confusion, because they are visual cues. Health professionals should consider the following when consulting with visually impaired children or young people.

➤ It is important to establish what type of visual impairment the young person experiences, as this will determine seating arrangements. It is necessary to sit within the child or young person's focal range and visual field. For example, for someone with peripheral vision and short focal range, the optimum seating position is close and to the side.

➤ Lighting levels are important. Where there is a source of natural light in the room, it is generally necessary to sit the child or young person with their back to the window to avoid visual glare.

➤ Auditory distractions need to be minimal. Usually, when someone is visually impaired, sound is their best distance sense, so they can be particularly distracted by auditory stimuli.

➤ Alerting through touch is often used with people who have a visual impairment but it is important to establish whether any tactile indicators or signals are needed. It is vital to be sensitive to where they do or do not want to be touched as there can be safeguarding issues involved. The shoulder is generally a safe area to touch prior to introducing yourself. Indeed, touch anywhere other than the shoulder, arm or hand should be avoided.

➤ It is helpful always to start each remark with the child or young person's name to ensure they are aware that you are addressing them in particular.

➤ Fatigue, time of day, and medications can cause fluctuating vision.

Learning disability

Learning disabilities are usually present from infancy and can shape both intellectual and social learning. A wide variety of skills may be affected, such as the ability to concentrate, remember or behave appropriately. In some instances, the (child or) young person's ability level may have been formally assessed and a psychological or school report summarises the nature of their difficulties. Health professionals might like to consider the following guidance.

➤ In general, it is useful to minimise distractions in the consultation setting. It can be helpful to have some toys available but too many can be overwhelming. Noisy toys should not be included as they can make it very difficult to hear what is being said. If a child or young person starts to use such a distraction it can create difficulty in discouraging them from carrying on.

➤ Gaining some idea of level of functioning from parents, carers and teachers is extremely useful to help know where to 'pitch' the level of communication with the child or young person. However, it is also important for the health professional to observe, and be alert to areas of competence and to adjust the level of communication accordingly.

➤ Making decisions about what is age or developmentally appropriate can be difficult. With young adults, there can be a tendency to infantilise, by giving soft toys for example. It is advisable to check if this is what the young person wants. For example, one young man with multiple difficulties, when given the opportunity to communicate on this topic, indicated that he did not want to be given soft toys any more. He wanted DVDs and other things that adolescents want.

➤ Be aware of sensory elements such as auditory and visual distractions which may influence the situation. Hunger, thirst and toileting needs may cause distractibility. Time of day can also have an influence, as (children and) young people can be very tired in the late afternoon.

Autistic spectrum disorder (ASD)

The three central difficulties experienced by children and young people with this condition are social communication, social interaction and imagination. Perhaps the most apparent manifestation of autism is the way in which it affects the person's ability to communicate with others. The spectrum refers to the fact that children and young people can be affected to various degrees, ranging from mild to extreme cases where social interaction is severely impaired. Individuals who are less affected can have relatively normal language and cognitive ability and this form of ASD is known as Asperger's syndrome. Typically, young people with autism have difficulty understanding subtle social clues in gesture and speech. They feel more comfortable with black and white rules rather than shades of grey. Speech is interpreted literally, so word play or sarcasm can be very confusing for them. Structure and predictability are very important in making them feel comfortable. Health professionals should consider the following as guidance.

➤ A quiet physical environment is very important to child or young people with ASD and distractions should be kept to a minimum. Loud noises can be very off-putting for them and curtains may have to be drawn to reduce extraneous sights and sounds.

➤ Positioning – it is generally better to allow the child or young person to choose where they want to sit and where they would like the other person to sit. If they have difficulty in exercising a choice, then ask permission to sit in your preferred position.

➤ Children or young people with ASD become extremely anxious and feel more comfortable with rules or guidelines that help them predict what is going to happen. They may like a specific list of stages of the session written down to enable them to refer to when needed. The format might be:
  — welcome
  — set-up session
  — drink
  — discussion
  — finish and arrange next meeting.

➤ They may need to know if follow-up meetings will be held at the same time, day and room.

➤ It can be very helpful to have specific signals such as a specific phrase or activity which lets them know that the session has begun and ended.

➤ Sensory issues can be particularly important for this group of people as they may feel the need to touch things while the session takes place. They may have their own object which satisfies their need to 'fiddle' but it is useful to have something available for this purpose, such as a stress ball or beanbag.

➤ Try not to be distracted by their 'twiddling' or 'rocking' behaviour if presented; this behaviour may be a comfort to them and help them deal with the anxiety of a new situation.

Hyperactivity and attention deficit hyperactivity disorder (ADHD)

Some children and young people find it very difficult to focus their attention for more than short periods and appear to be very active or impulsive. They may seem forgetful and disorganised and such behaviour can appear to be rude and uncaring. In some cases this is an extension of normal behaviour and it can be made more obvious by excessive intake of sugar or caffeine. Home circumstances may also be contributory as they may be acting out anxieties about home life or they may not have experienced consistent parenting, which would help them develop good attention skills. In its most extreme form, the child or young person may be judged to have attention deficit hyperactivity disorder (ADHD). Health professionals might like to consider the following.

➤ Consultations with hyperactive children and young people can be really challenging and can quickly result in chaos without some degree of planning. General principles which have been shown to be effective should be applied. These include reducing obvious distractions, creating a calm environment and maintaining a calm and warm disposition. Giving clear, consistent but firm directions is helpful as is providing lots of positive feedback and maintaining a sense of humour.

➤ In addition to reducing distractions for this group, it is also important to pay attention to the temperature in the room. Some children and young people are not good at recognising when they are too hot and the adult may have to check with them if they are getting too hot or cold.

➤ Children and young people with ADHD may find it difficult to sit down for too long and may need to have little breaks to walk around.

➤ Younger children may get rather excited and in these instances those who are especially over-responsive to stimulation may benefit from an activity which provides proprioceptive feedback. This is feedback in their body from an activity that stimulates their muscles and helps them determine their 'position in space'. It can help them become calmer. A 'Space Hopper', a large rubber ball with handles that the child can sit on and bounce in place, can be useful for this purpose.

➤ Using the person's name frequently can be helpful in focusing their attention and allows them to recognise that you are talking to them.

Cerebral palsy

Cerebral palsy is the term which is used to describe a physical impairment that affects movement. The movement problems vary from very mild to extremely severe and vary widely from one individual to another. There are three main types, which correspond to injuries to different parts of the brain:

1. Children and young people with **spastic** cerebral palsy have muscles that become very stiff and weak, especially under effort. This can affect their control of movement.
2. Children and young people with **athetoid** cerebral palsy have some loss of control of their posture, and they tend to make unwanted movements.
3. Children and young people with **ataxic** cerebral palsy usually have problems with balance and may also have shaky hand movements and irregular speech.

Health professionals might like to consider the following guidance.

➤ Distractions are to be avoided as sudden noises, for example, can make them startle and cause them to go into spasm.

➤ Visual impairment may be present and this needs to be taken into consideration in terms of lighting and positioning.

➤ Positioning and comfort can be significant in this condition and this should be checked regularly. 'Wobble cushions' (small inflatable cushions) may aid with this issue.

➤ Fatigue can set in easily for a number of reasons. The effort of maintaining position and communicating can be extremely tiring. In addition, the child or young person may be on a cocktail of medication which can make them lethargic.

➤ Heat, thirst and toileting needs can be issues and should be checked to ensure comfort.

➤ If the child or young person has speech this may be indistinct. If this means you have difficulty in understanding, it is better to ask for clarification than to pretend to understand. You can seek help from the child, young person and accompanying adult by asking them to help you understand. Recognise that you are new to the person and you have to learn about their communication. Breath control is often difficult for people with cerebral palsy and it can help if they are encouraged to slow their speech down.

More detailed information about an extremely wide range of conditions can be found from Contact a Family. This organisation provides support, advice and information for families with disabled children and young people. Their web address is: www.cafamily.org.uk.

Wheelchair etiquette

People who use wheelchairs comment that at times they can feel invisible. People talk to those who accompany them about them, rather than to them directly. The assumption can be perceived to be that if someone is in a wheelchair they may be intellectually impaired also. They can feel at a disadvantage because eye contact can be more difficult to achieve.

- Be aware of the needs of the wheelchair user before they come into the room to avoid making them uncomfortable by chairs having to be rearranged or access being restricted.
- When talking to someone in a wheelchair, where possible, do so at eye level.
- Be aware about invading their personal space – do not lean on their chair for example.
- Ask if help is required rather than assuming that it is.
- Young people in wheelchairs will need transfers for washrooms and transportation. When transfers occur, don't move the wheelchair out of reach from the child. Keep it in close proximity.

FORMALISED COMMUNICATION METHODS

Where children and young people have severe problems with communication, highly specialised techniques may have been devised at home and within educational setting to build on the child or young person's communication abilities. These will have been the result of many hours' skilled and patient teaching. Thus, it is important for the health professional to understand, respect and use these in the consultation to help the child or young person participate as fully as possible. Seeking advice about the system of communication to be used can be helpful to the health professional in terms of learning about the child or young person's ability generally as well as in terms of communication skills. This process is also helpful in establishing rapport and provides an opportunity to observe an 'expert' carer demonstrating how they interact and include the child or young person in discussion.

Many children and young people with special needs will use alternative and augmentative communication methods. These can range from voice output devices to multisensory references and will depend entirely on the individual's physical and cognitive abilities. This will have been assessed, usually at school, and a method or device chosen which is developmentally appropriate given all the factors involved. Children learn first through the senses and thus those who have impairment in any of these are at a disadvantage in learning. They may be helped by prompting using one or more of the methods outlined below.

Multisensory references are usually for children and young people with visual or dual-sensory impairment. They can range from a basic cup and spoon to indicate food and drink to a variety of tactile, auditory or olfactory elements to indicate location, time or people. For example, wearing the same perfume or aftershave can help the child or young person recognise who you are by building up an association with that scent over time.

Photographs, pictures and symbols are used for non-verbal children and young people with good visual acuity. Children and young people have to learn to interpret information contained in photographs but once successful with photographs of familiar objects, people and places, this skill can be extended to photographs of unfamiliar objects, people and places. This is followed by progression on to printed pictures and then to symbols such as Makaton. These images can build into a communication board or book, which is normally accessed via eye-pointing or targeting with the hand, foot or a pointer, or by verbal facilitation from a helper.

These 'low-tech' methods can be transferred to more 'high-tech' devices, such as GoTalk, or MessageMate, or devices from the DynaVox range (*see* Figure 10.1a), all

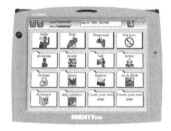 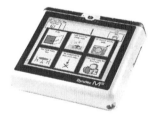

FIGURE 10.1A DynaVox range

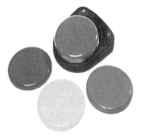

FIGURE 10.1B BIGmack

of which allow images to be accessed but, when targeted, result in a pre-recorded word or message being spoken.

The simplest of all voice output devices is the single-message switch, the BIGmack (*see* Figure 10.1b). This allows a pre-recorded message to be played when the switch is pressed, thus giving the young person some control through speech, with messages such as, 'I need to go to the toilet'.

Other devices allow more complicated use of recorded speech but depend on greater recognition of a range of pictures and symbols and a greater degree of accuracy in activating the switches.

Computer-based communication systems are plentiful and can be accessed via single switches, adapted keyboards, mouse, or even sound recognition. If the child or young person has a communication system it is essential and respectful to address them and not to talk through the accompanying adult. This is only appropriate when additional guidance is required.

Signing and symbols

Signing and symbols are not only used for communicating with the hearing impaired, but also to augment other communication systems. British Sign Language and Makaton are the most common signing systems; Makaton is the most popular and most appropriate for children and young people with severe and complex needs. Widgit Software also produces a large range of materials using symbols to aid inclusion.

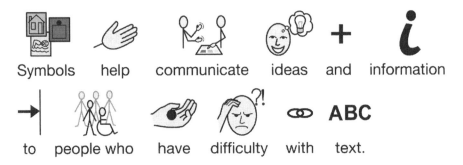

FIGURE 10.2 Widgit Symbols © Widgit Software 2010, www.widgit.com

Signing can be used to indicate key words in a sentence, such as 'you' and 'car', while actually saying, 'Did you come in the car today?' Be prepared for the child or young person not to be able to sign back due to fine- and gross-motor difficulties, but they may respond by indicating yes or no.

COMMUNICATING WITH CHILDREN AND YOUNG PEOPLE WITH SEVERE LEARNING DIFFICULTIES

On first meeting, introductions and outlining the purpose of the meeting are necessary as well as ascertaining any other issues the child or young person, parent and

COMMUNICATION CHALLENGES **161**

health professional want to discuss. Acknowledge that it may take longer for an unfamiliar person to communicate with the child or young person. This clarifies the position for the child or young person and over time improves as trust and confidence is established. If communication is limited this is an ideal time to clarify and ask for a demonstration by using a few test questions.

➤ Make it clear that as a health professional you do not necessarily know what issues the child or young person might like to discuss.
➤ If they are shy or have significant communication problems, it can be helpful to suggest that the parent accompanying them begins if the child or young person agrees.
➤ Suggest that the child or young person can indicate if they do not agree with what their parent is saying and then they will get their chance to talk about it.
➤ Sit opposite the child or young person and beside the parent, to ensure that you are paying attention to them primarily and the parent second.
➤ Confidentiality – should be explained simply and briefly. If there is anything which you feel needs to be shared with other people then this would be discussed. For example, parents might not be told everything that the child or young person has disclosed if they have stated that they do not wish this to happen – unless of course the disclosure reveals a safeguarding issue.

Possible outline for 'difficult' consultations

After the initial consultation matters have been addressed, it may be time to examine challenging issues such as behaviour. This is a suggested outline for beginning this conversation.

➤ Prompt: 'Is there something you would like to talk to us about?'
➤ Prompt the parent to provide a positive description of the child or young person's abilities, interests and characteristics.
➤ Reinforce the positive attributes and then mention things that you would like to speak to them about, such as behaviour problems.
➤ 'We think that you may be unhappy about something and that makes you [bite your lip]. We would like to find out if there is something we can do to help that so you do not need to [bite your lip] anymore.'
➤ Observe reaction closely.
➤ 'Is that right?'

The child or young person's communication ability at this point is the key to how you proceed. If they only have a yes and no, then closed questions providing forced choices will be required. For example, 'Are you unhappy about something at school? Home?', and so on. Care should always be taken to check that you are getting things right by reflecting things back to the child or young person and others present. Where the child or young person has a more formalised communication system, for example a communication book, then more options can be presented: 'Do you want to talk about feelings, people, food?' Then go through the options on the page indicated. For some children and young people, processing this information and producing a response can take some time. It is important not to interrupt and ask the question again too quickly as the child or young person will have to start processing this from the beginning. It is common for communication to take a long time and cannot be hurried.

This can be a very emotional session for all concerned. The child or young person may demonstrate relief that someone is recognising an area of difficulty and is willing to offer help. For the professional, it can be difficult to balance professional detachment and human emotion as some topics which the child or young person wants to discuss can be challenging. Also, the process can be tiring for all concerned. A parent might be surprised by the extent to which the child or young person is able to express their own feelings when given the opportunity.

Given the reasons, means and opportunity, the child or young person is helped through the process of discussion and dialogue and in our experience may communicate about many of the issues which are relevant to most children or young people. The following examples are drawn from sessions which began as described above. All of the children or young people described had severe forms of cerebral palsy and were wheelchair users. All had significant problems with speech although a few could produce one or two words if sufficiently relaxed – not usually the case when talking about problem areas. All had been taught to indicate yes or no in a way which was appropriate for their areas of control. This could be a smile for 'yes' and a downturned mouth for 'no'; it could be eye-pointing to hand, right for 'yes' left for 'no'; or it could be different sounds for yes and no.

In these sessions, the psychologist was the visiting health professional and she worked together with the teacher and where possible the parent, thus at times there was a four-way consultation. In order to make this workable, we followed certain patterns in all sessions. We worked in a quiet room where there were few distractions. The child or young person sat in their chair and the other people sat in an arc in front of the child or young person. The teacher, as the familiar person, introduced the psychologist to the child or young person and to the parent, if present. The teacher then outlined the purpose of the meeting, which was taking place because it was believed that the child or young person was unhappy about things. If we could talk about this, we might find out how to make things a little better for the child or young person. The psychologist would introduce her contribution by explaining that she meets lots of children and talks about difficulties with them.

This was an opportunity for the psychologist to explain that she was not yet familiar with the child or young person's communication system. The teacher explains the communication system and the child or young person demonstrates how to use it. The topics for discussion were behaviours at school or at home, which had given rise to the belief that there was a problem, and these were described by the teacher or parent, as appropriate. The child or young person's reaction (agitation, looking sad, etc.) then gave us the feedback to ask closed questions to refine the nature of the problem. Great care was taken to ensure that we were interpreting the child or young person's views correctly, by checking throughout that what we were expressing for them was what they meant. The psychologist was then able to contextualise the problem and suggest strategies for tackling it. This was then negotiated with the child or young person and a further meeting was arranged to review progress and discuss further issues. The children or young people used the sessions very well and reacted positively to them. The sessions were very time-consuming and exhausting for all concerned but the children or young people showed considerable behaviour change in response to this approach as can be seen from the following examples.

Sibling rivalry

Mary (11) who lived at a residential school indicated (by means of a symbol communication book) that she was angry with her brother, who also had a disability but lived at home with their parents. In particular, she wanted to have her mother's attention at bedtime when she was at home and also wished her brother, who was younger, would go to bed before her. She appeared to be relieved to learn that most brothers and sisters can feel angry with one another and that this is not disloyal. She listened attentively and with apparent relief to simple examples about other children who showed the same feelings. This helped contextualise her feelings as normal. Her mother was able to respond to this knowledge by changing the bedtime routine when Mary was at home.

Following this, Mary was much happier and more settled at night. Her issue about being at school while her brother was at home could not be resolved but through time she came to accept the reasons for this in terms of their different needs. By picking up on the fact that Mary frequently had difficulty getting off to sleep at school and discussing this with her, she was able to communicate that she found it hard to get to sleep in one position and wanted to change. The teacher agreed to discuss this with the nurse and physiotherapist and they were able to allow her to fall asleep in her preferred position. Following this change, Mary was much more settled at night and was able to express her happiness about this outcome in subsequent sessions.

Anger management

John (10) attends a residential special school. He was referred as he was exhibiting behaviours such as shouting, screaming, self-harm (hitting his forehead with his fist) and reaching out to harm others in the classroom and at home and at school. Through a series of questions with yes and no responses we were able to ascertain that John was behaving in this way because he wanted food. Working with his family informed us that his parents tended to indulge him when he behaved in this way by immediately giving him snacks or meals. Subsequent sessions helped John to understand the need to wait and that food would be offered to him at the appropriate times. The key to this success was consistency of approach by the staff at the school and in the residential setting as well as within the family home and the fact that this approach had been explained to and negotiated with John rather than just implemented.

Food presentation

In discussing issues about food another student, Paul (12), indicated that he liked to see his food before it was cut up for him. The teacher communicated this to other staff and as a result the usual policy of presenting food to students was changed. It was evident from other students' responses to this change that this was a popular decision. This helped to emphasise the importance of choice for this group of young people as with other young people. It was a topic which was repeated with other students with regard to choice in the clothes they wear, how their bedrooms are decorated and the type of presents they like to receive.

Involvement in decision-making

The mother of Peter (10) explained that he had not been happy on his weekend at home. He kept shouting out at night and would not settle. She commented that she could not understand it because his bedroom was lovely as it had recently been decorated. Peter reacted through posturing and vocalisation at this point, prompting further discussion about the decoration of his bedroom. This revealed that he was not happy with the decor as he felt it was too young for him. His mother acknowledged that she had not involved him in the decisions about this, although she was used to giving him choices about other aspects of his life. She decided to redecorate and this time she gave Peter an active role in this and more peaceful nights returned.

Bereavement issues

It is a sad fact of life that children and young people will experience bereavement. Children and young people with disabilities are more likely to experience loss than those without disabilities or illness. We have come across several examples where children or young people have been upset by the loss of a family member or a friend but we have discovered that no one has then spoken to them about this. One young man who was new to the school had recently lost his mother. As staff had not known her they were reluctant to raise the issue with him. In a session, we gave him the opportunity to discuss his loss and introduced the topic by making reference to the photo of his mother beside his bed. We asked him if he wanted to discuss this and he indicated yes. He also indicated that he did not want to discuss this at school but at home with his Dad. We were able to support his father in having this difficult discussion with his son. He also seemed relieved that this had been brought up. After this had taken place, this boy was able to indicate to staff, by looking at the photograph, when he wanted to talk about his mother.

Toileting

Rahim (14) had become so upset that he began to withdraw from all cooperation. He stopped using his signboard, stopped eating and stopped indicating his toileting needs. Once he had begun to engage in sessions where we explored what was making him unhappy, we were able to talk about toileting. We explained that he did not need to show us that he was unhappy by withdrawal as we were aware of why he was unhappy. We requested that he indicate when he needed to go to the toilet once more. He responded positively.

Self-harm

By discussing with Mary that she no longer needed to bite her lip to express her frustration, she was able to reduce the extent to which she used a self-harm strategy, even though this had become a long-standing problem.

Food control

It is not uncommon for children and young people with complex needs to express some of their difficulties through their response to food as it one area where they can exercise some control. This can be evident in behaviour such as food refusal or spitting it out. Susan (14), who usually had someone to assist with her feeding, became noisy and uncooperative at mealtimes and appeared to be pushing the person away. This was expressed to her and she was given an opportunity to hold the spoon herself, although she could not maintain this throughout a whole mealtime. With discussion about the level of help which might be acceptable, she was able to enjoy more independence with this activity and accept a minimum level of help. Although this was messy, she fed well and it appeared to give her a sense of achievement and raised self-esteem.

Comparison with children/young people without disabilities

The range of issues which these young people express has been strikingly similar to those expressed by other children young people who do not have the same physical challenges. These young people have raised with us issues relating to relationship with parents, who they sit with or who they live with in a residential house. Where they spend their leisure time, fairness and turn-taking and what clothes they wear are just as important to them. We have also found that children and young people with severe difficulties of movement and little or no speech have been able to make use of a range of techniques which are useful with most other children.

Relaxation/visualisation

John (11) was an anxious boy with cerebral palsy who would become hot and sweaty when most apprehensive and, as a consequence, thirsty and distracted. He was given the opportunity to use visualisation techniques through a story-telling model. He was taught relaxation skills, breathing and muscle relaxation as well as thinking about his favourite place. His favourite place turned out to be somewhere snowy and he imagined playing outside. This had the visible effect of controlling his mood and his anxiety, which consequently reduced his temperature and thirst enabling him to continue to discuss other issues he wanted to share.

Social story

This is an established technique using a personalised story with or without pictures to demonstrate a situation or event which is new, unfamiliar or upsetting to the child or young person. Louise (9) was due to go to hospital for an ultrasound appointment. She was always anxious about hospital appointments and procedures. The staff at the residential school were able to help Louise prepare for this by introducing the social story, 'Arnold has an ultrasound', before her visit which illustrated a fictional character going to hospital for the same procedure. In the story, the child's questions were answered and coping strategies described.

Such stories or discussions with others assist the normalisation process, by helping them to understand that other children and young people feel as they do and that this is 'normal'. Children and young people with special needs often have limited opportunity for such learning because of their limitations in verbal communication and also because much of the talk directed to them concerns their immediate physical needs.

The difficulties that these children and young people can experience and the limitations they face are usually evident. This can lead us to make assumptions about their lack of ability to communicate. However, our experience has shown that many are able to express their feelings, wishes and needs when given the appropriate time, space and support personal to them. The underlying assumption should be that all children and young people can communicate and have the right to do so. It is our responsibility as parents and professionals to ensure that they are given the tools to release their potential.

I am the child

I am the child who cannot talk. You often pity me; I see it in your eyes. You wonder how much I am aware of – I see that as well. I am aware of much – whether you are happy or sad or fearful, patient or impatient, full of love and desire, or if you are just doing your duty by me. I marvel at your frustration, knowing mine to be far greater, for I cannot express myself or my needs as you do.

You cannot conceive my isolation, so complete it is at times. I do not gift you with clever conversation, cute remarks to be laughed over and repeated. I do not give you answers to your everyday questions, responses over my well-being, sharing my needs, or comments about the world about me. I do not give you rewards as defined by the world's standards – great strides in development that you can credit yourself; I do not give you understanding as you know it.

What I give you is so much more valuable – I give you instead opportunities. Opportunities to discover the depth of your character, not mine; the depth of your love, your commitment, your patience, your abilities; the opportunity to explore your spirit more deeply than you imagined possible. I drive you further than you would ever go on your own, working harder, seeking answers to your many questions with no answers. I am the child who cannot talk.

I am the child who cannot walk. The world seems to pass me by. You see the longing in my eyes to get out of this chair, to run and play like other children. There is much you take for granted. I want the toys on the shelf, I need to go to the bathroom, oh I've dropped my fork again. I am dependent on you in these ways. My gift to you is to make you more aware of your great fortune, your healthy back and legs, your ability to do for yourself. Sometimes people appear not to notice me; I always notice them. I feel not so much envy as desire;

desire to stand upright, to put one foot in front of the other, to be independent. I give you awareness. I am the child who cannot walk.

I am the child who is mentally impaired. I don't learn easily, if you judge me by the world's measuring stick, what I do know is infinite joy in simple things. I am not burdened as you are with the strifes and conflicts of a more complicated life. My gift to you is to grant you the freedom to enjoy things as a child, to teach you how much your arms around me mean, to give you love. I give you the gift of simplicity. I am the child who is mentally impaired.

I am the disabled child. I am your teacher. If you allow me, I will teach you what is really important in life. I will give you and teach you unconditional love. I gift you with my innocent trust, my dependency upon you. I teach you about how precious this life is and about not taking things for granted. I teach you about forgetting your own needs and desires and dreams. I teach you giving. Most of all I teach you hope and faith. I am the disabled child. (Author unknown)

REFERENCES

1 United Nations. *Convention on the Rights of the Child*. New York: United Nations; 1990. General Assembly resolution 44/25 of 20 November 1989; entry into force 2 September 1990. Available at: http://treaties.un.org/Pages/ViewDetails.aspx?src=TREATY&mtdsg_no=IV-11&chapter=4&lang=en (accessed 20 June 2010).
2 Department of Health and Social Security (DHSS, now defunct). *Fit for the Future: report of the Committee on Child Health Services* (Court Report). London: HMSO; 1976.
3 Office of Public Sector Information (OPSI). *Disability Discrimination Act 2005*. London: OPSI; 2005. Available at: www.opsi.gov.uk/Acts/acts2005/ukpga_20050013_en_1 (accessed 20 June 2010).
4 Department of Children, Schools and Families, Department of Health. *Aiming High for Disabled Children (AHDC)*. London: DH; 2007. Available at: www.dcsf.gov.uk/everychild matters/healthandwellbeing/ahdc/AHDC/ (accessed 20 June 2010).
5 White-Koning M, Arnaud C, Dickinson HO, Thyen U, *et al.* Determinants of child–parent agreement in quality-of-life reports: a European study of children with cerebral palsy. *Pediatrics*. 2007; **120**; e804–e814.

CHAPTER 11

Taking your child to a consultation: the parents' perspective

Pippa Hemingway

INTRODUCTION

Parents play a crucial part in the success or failure of child involvement in decision-making about their healthcare. This is as true for an acutely ill child as for children with chronic conditions. This chapter is set within an emergency care context, as an emergency department (ED) must accommodate the needs of children and accompanying families as far as reasonably possible.[1] Although the evidence relating to emergency care consultations and child participation in decision-making is sparse, it is a crucial setting because of the often serious nature of the illnesses or injuries experienced by children. The evidence relating to parents within emergency care and from the wider literature pertaining to parental perspectives and roles as both passive recipients and active role models within child consultations is presented in this chapter. Two methods of preparation of children by parents and parental modelling are discussed. Parents may use such methods to facilitate and support their children to take part in decision-making at a high level of participation and to encourage child and parental communication within consultations with health professionals. The chapter ends with a guide for parents' incorporating 12 questions that a parent may wish to consider prior to attending a consultation with a child, to maximise the level of child participation.

Chapter 2 focused on consultations with children suffering from chronic illness. The context for the current chapter is the child or young person with an acute illness or injury with particular reference to those seen in the ED. Many parents will relate to the ED either through their own experience of attending (with or without a child) or by watching television programmes such as *Casualty* and *ER*. The information for parents and health professionals in this chapter is also useful to those attending, managing and caring for children in primary care settings such as the GP surgery,

GP out-of-hours service and unscheduled care locations such as walk-in centres and minor injury units. However, parents seen in any healthcare location should find this chapter of use with some tailoring to their particular child's healthcare needs. Clearly, for reasons of patient safety, for those parents with children with life-threatening or severe illness or injury the opportunities for active roles in the consultation may be reduced until the child is stabilised.

PARENTS' AND CHILDREN'S VOICES IN THE EMERGENCY DEPARTMENT

In the UK, the health professionals that a parent and child may encounter during their ED attendance may be hospital doctors, GPs, nurses, emergency care practitioners, phlebotomists, radiographers, play specialists and liaison health visitors, to name a few. The number and range of health professionals presents the parent with multiple opportunities to encourage active child consultation with some or all of the health professionals that they may meet in the ED.

Evidence relating to health professional and child communication in the UK is scarce within an emergency care setting and beyond. However, a study from the US is available, although the context differs from the UK NHS healthcare system. Wissow *et al.* (1998) examined patient–provider communication during the emergency care of children with asthma.[2] They conducted a cross-sectional, observational study which examined 104 children aged 4–9 years and their guardian(s) attending emergency departments in seven cities in the US. They found that within the emergency department, although providers' talk to children was largely supportive and directive, child talk was minimal (an average of 20 child statements per visit versus 156 by parents). The authors concluded that children took little part in discussions during their emergency asthma care and that conversation should be directed towards both parents and children.[2] Alberti (2007) reported in the period 2005–6 that 98% of patients were seen, diagnosed and treated within four hours of arrival at ED.[3] However, the current four-hour waiting-time target in ED is facing revision in line with clinical evidence which, although the full implications are as yet unclear, should provide opportunity for active child consultation with a wide range of health professionals.

Furthermore, the majority of consultations in UK EDs are initiated by parents. Bradley *et al.* (1995) examined the source of referral of children brought to a children's ED and those consulting their GP over a six-week period in the inner city of Belfast. They reported that 82% of children were referred by parents directly without consulting other health professionals prior to arriving at the ED.[4] Parents who seek consultation in the ED on their own may already be empowered and encouraged to maintain this active role once in the ED. Parents may promote their children's voices to be heard within the consultations taking place while in the department and within those that follow (for example, follow-up ED attendance, GP surgery attendance). A further study found that 46% of parents attend the ED with children suffering from minor illness to obtain self-care advice.[5] Parents require advice about how to care for the child with a specific illness or injury (and how children may take care of themselves in an age-appropriate manner) and this provides good opportunities for active participation in ED consultations.

A Scottish Executive policy document recommends that all emergency care practitioners should actively involve children and young people in their care and treatment. It points out that involvement in decision-making encourages feelings of control in a child, increases confidence and helps in the treatment and recovery process.[6] In addition, the Intercollegiate Committee for Services for Children in Emergency Departments recommends that EDs must accommodate the needs of children and accompanying families as far as reasonably possible.[1] While not stipulating active participation in decision-making by children directly, it is clear that the needs of children incorporate such involvement in consultations in the ED.

PARENTAL PERSPECTIVES ON CONSULTATIONS

Parents, when asked to describe their ideal consultation with a child, made the following points.[7]

➤ A focus on the whole person: parents wanted a treatment provider to focus on the whole person not just the presenting illness or injury.
➤ A welcoming and relaxed atmosphere: the provider should be welcoming and show a sincere interest in the child and situation; the provider should be able to make the child relax and gain confidence.
➤ Enough time: parents wanted sufficient time to talk freely about the child's illness.
➤ Questions and elaborations: parents wanted to be asked questions about their child's symptoms and problems and how the child's environment might be affecting the problems.
➤ Explanation and information: parents wished for explanations and information on what the cause of the problem could be, what the symptoms might be connected to, how treatment was going to work, and about the expectations for the treatment results.

These themes arose from a small qualitative interview study with parents of 16 children aged 0–10 years undertaken in Norway.[7] While this study examined parental perspectives of consultations with doctors and homeopaths rather than with ED health professionals, it suggests that parents have an important perspective to offer to the consultation process. The five themes outlined may transfer to UK healthcare settings.

Parents report that UK primary care consultations about children are challenging. Many parents find it difficult to decide when to consult: they do not wish to appear overanxious; they worry about insufficient consultation length; they are concerned about feeling dismissed or 'fobbed off'; they have problems understanding medical jargon and are anxious about the health professional failing to identify their main concerns.[8] Clearly there may be a discrepancy between the parental perceptions of the ideal consultation and reality. The box below presents an example of how to improve a child's experience of being in the ED.

> ### Hearing a child's voice in the emergency department
>
> Henry is a seven-year-old boy who, after falling from his bike, has sustained an abrasion to his elbow, which is ingrained with grit. Henry has been assessed by the doctor in the ED and has been told that the abrasion needs cleaning prior to dressing. Within the treatment room, his mother, Rachel, is also with him. A play specialist works in the department and is also present in the treatment room. She asks Henry if he wants to play while his wound is cleaned and dressed (as well as when the doctor injects local anaesthetic). Rachel asks Henry to tell the play specialist what he wants to decide. Henry tells the play specialist that he does not know what to do and he is given a range of play choices. He chooses some verbal games to play, facilitated by the play specialist and his mother while his wound is cleaned and dressed (distraction therapy). He does notice the wound being cleaned but feels more in control and he reports that it didn't hurt much.

In this example, it would have been easy for the parent to speak for her child and make the decision herself but she allowed him to make his own decisions. This increased Henry's control over a potentially fearful situation and reduced his anxiety, which has in turn been shown to reduce the experience of pain.[9] Play therapy can be a vital adjunct in preparing children for painful and invasive procedures within the ED environment. Goymour *et al.* (2000) define that play therapy provides developmentally appropriate distraction to facilitate the child's coping strategies throughout hospital examinations and procedures.[9]

There are various levels of child participation and this example is aligned to Shier's model of children's participation at Level 4, where the child is involved in decision-making processes.[10] Shier's model was originally intended to assist health professionals to identify at which level they are at currently in their own practice and what the next steps are to increase children's participation.[11] The two aspects (levels and openings) could be used by parents to choose a level of participation they wish to encourage within a particular consultation.

Shier's model of children's participation[10,11]

Levels of participation*	Openings
5. Children share power and responsibility for decision-making.	Are you ready to share some of your adult power with children?
4. Children are involved in decision-making processes.	Are you ready to let children join in (the) decision-making processes?
3. Children's views are taken into account.	Are you ready to take children's views into account?

Levels of participation*	Openings
2. Children are supported in expressing their views.	Are you ready to support your children in expressing their views?
1. Children are listened to.	Are you ready to listen to children?

* Higher participation levels are represented by higher numbers.

This section has introduced the concept of a parent encouraging child participation within the consultation. The next section expands on the idea that active parental participation is required, as opposed to adoption of passive roles, if we are to hear the potential of children's and young people's voices within their consultations.

PARENTAL ROLES IN CONSULTATION

Passive role

The traditional view of healthcare delivery involved a power imbalance between the professional and the patient. The health professional was viewed as all-powerful during the consultation, the consultation was on their terms and was guided by the questions they asked.[12] The child was observed to be a passive participant during the consultation.[13] In some clinical areas this model still prevails. Wissow *et al.* (1998) suggest that the majority of consulting statements within the emergency department are biomedical and are led by the health professional.[2] Another more recent study reported, when describing and assessing components of doctor–parent–child communication in an outpatient setting, that doctors contributed most to the conversation, conducting 61% of the audio-taped conversation with children being heard to speak for only 4% of the consultation.[14] Rylance (2004) concluded that the participation of children needs to be encouraged as part of a child-centred approach. Chapter 2 addresses parental factors influential in their key role in consultations with their child and health professional. It is of interest here to examine the studies mentioned above for the amount of parental participation. Rylance (2004) reported that parents' communication overwhelmingly focused on giving information (83% of their recorded voice), seeking information (13% of their recorded voice) or social conversation (4% of their recorded voice). The absence of the parental voice in encouraging the child to actively participate is noticeable. The parents most likely assumed a passive role in the consultation and we may presume that any child participation might have been led by the health professional in the consultation. Wissow *et al.* (1998) reported in their study that parents made 156 statements versus 20 statements made by the child towards the health professional, which suggests that parents were less passive than children in their patient–provider communication in the emergency care environment.[2] However, parents talked to children via only 57 statements indicating low levels of communication to children. This suggests that parents were passive in their direct encouragement of child participation within the consultation; however, the extent to which the 57 statements related to empowering the child to participate was not reported.

The complexity of parental encouragement

Parental involvement cannot be seen as a clear-cut involved/not involved dichotomy. Several factors indicate that the choice to facilitate child involvement remains flexible and varies depending on the precise situation. A study by Runeson *et al.* (2002) found that even at higher levels of participation parents sometimes follow a passive role in the presence of health professionals. The parents rarely questioned anything or entered into a conversation when the professionals were present. However, when the professional was absent the parent asked what the child thought and supported him or her in making a decision.[15] This study highlights that the parental role may vary between active enquirer and passive recipient of information regarding the child's health depending on the health professionals' presence. However, it may not be the parents' fault that they do not take an active role in encouraging the child to participate fully in the consultations. Wissow and Kimel (2002) outlined the barriers to communication in the ED include noise, anxiety, confusion and differences in language and expectations.[16] In addition, it is well known that intercultural differences can have marked consequences for healthcare of children.[17] Clearly external factors create a barrier to parents promoting an active role for their children, while some barriers can arise from internal factors. Within the ED environment a key internal factor may be that some parents feel that the mental burden of taking complicated decisions should be left to themselves, especially when their children are coping with illness, injury or are in the process of being hospitalised.[18] This concurs with the perception that participation may need to be adapted or halted when the child's condition is life-threatening or sudden deterioration requires medical help.

Active roles

The box below outlines young people's descriptions of five active roles that parents perform in communication in the setting of potentially life-threatening chronic illness.[19]

Young people's descriptions of the roles parents performed in communication[19]

- Facilitators of communication between health professionals and themselves: for example, the parent's presence in consultations sometimes gives the child confidence to ask questions.
- Envoys: for example, when young people brief their parents to seek information on their behalf.
- Communication buffers: for example, when young people used their parents to shield them from the burden of answering questions.
- Human databases: when parents acted as cataloguers and repositories of information about the illness.
- Communication brokers: when parents customised, clarified or reiterated information so that young people could better assimilate what health professionals had said.

While the setting differs from the ED acute setting, the roles stipulated by Young *et al.* (2003) may remain relevant to parents in the ED setting attending with acutely ill children and for those children attending the ED with unstable chronic illness.[19,20] It is clear that many of these parental roles are active but they also in part allow the child to remain passive in their involvement when the child wishes. A recent review of decision-support needs of parents making child health decisions suggests that although parents desire information from health professionals they are often reluctant to ask questions and to challenge the health professionals' authority, especially if that view is perceived to differ from their own.[21] The role of 'human database' may be assisted by parents being provided with (or seeking) written information in advance of a consultation with a health professional and this may prepare parents to ask more questions within the consultation.[21] The active role of being a 'human database' and the other roles indicated by Young *et al.* (2003) should not be mistaken with privileged parental accounts.[19,22] This is where health professionals affirm the parent as the best person to communicate information concerning their children at the expense of marginalising the children's role so they withdraw from the consultation.[22]

Active methods

Parents may now be more willing to encourage their children to participate in paediatric consultations than in the past.[23] Having a voice in decision-making gives parents a feeling that they are part of the team giving their child optimal care.[24] Parents have a significant influence on whether children's efforts to participate are facilitated and supported in the hospital setting.[25] To fulfil an active role, parents can use a variety of methods to prime the child to fully participate in decision-making when this is in the child's best interests so that the parent can become more involved in the communication regarding their child's health. Two key methods are preparation and parental modelling. Parents can use techniques, or 'little tricks' as they may perceive them, to encourage positive child behaviour. A parent hopefully will prepare a child that they need to go to hospital to attend ED before they set off and, once in the ED, act in a manner that they want the child to behave. These two methods are described more fully below, within the context of the ED.

PREPARATION

Over the time of parenthood, most parents will catch themselves saying something to their child along the lines of, 'Now, Charlotte, I need to take you to Grandma's this afternoon as Mummy has to go to the gym. I won't be long and I'll pick you up at teatime'. Or, 'In a couple of minutes I want you to pull the plug in the bath and then you need to dry yourself and get ready for bed'. The parent says this before the event described, in a process of preparing the child for what will happen next. The child needs to understand and to develop a mental framework for what is happening next and if the child, however young, fails in this she will experience anxiety and fear of events about to unfold.[26] Therefore, parents may recognise that children behave much better if they are prepared as the need for security is high in the hierarchy of basic human needs.[27] This time-honoured parental technique can be used by adapting it to prepare children for active participation in consultations with a health professional. Some parents may think that the urgency of taking a child to the ED will mean that this type of preparation is not possible. However, such preparation becomes even more vital when introducing a child, maybe for the first time, to the ED. It is recognised that there is a need to minimise pain, fear and anxiety in children presenting to the ED.[28] Only by doing so does an opportunity for parental facilitation of the child's involvement become possible.

Of equal importance is the need to prepare the child for its own involvement in healthcare decision-making processes. The optimal time for preparation is when the child is at home, as it has been shown that the extent to which children are encouraged by their parents to take routine responsibility for health maintenance tasks or having medications prescribed will in turn have a bearing on the nature of the encounter. This also affects the extent to which the parent seeks to speak on their behalf and the child's willingness to take an active part in the consultation and their subsequent compliance with whatever is decided.[23] However, if this is not possible time will usually be available, unless the child is severely ill or injured or the ED is unusually quiet, for preparation once the child has arrived at the department in the waiting time between initial assessment and medical consultation with a doctor or other emergency care practitioner. If some preparation is conducted at home or during routine appointments with the GP, for example, the time required for the parent to prepare the child for active participation in consultation may be less in more stressful situations.

PARENTAL MODELLING

The way the parent behaves in a consultation is central to how well the child will participate in the consultation at that time or in the future. To use a basic example which many parents may recognise, when a young child sees a spider for the first time, if the parent adopts fearful behaviour of the spider then the child will copy the parent and display the same fearful behaviour. This powerful effect is reinforced by a study by Gerull and Rapee (2002) who investigated the influence of parental modelling on the acquisition of fear and avoidance in toddler-age children. The 30 children were shown a rubber snake and rubber spider which were alternatively paired with either negative or positive facial expressions by their mothers. These authors found that the children showed greater fear expressions and avoidance of the stimuli following negative reactions from their mothers.[29] This may be used as an analogy for the consultation process. For example, a parent may choose to display positive behaviour in the consultation, actively asking questions that the child wants answers to, discussing the child's illness proactively, asking for alternatives to be considered and modelling the behaviour of someone who wants to be involved in the decision-making process. Even if the child does not want to participate at a high level on that day or with a certain health professional, the parent can 'model' the desired behaviour for the child, allowing for the required flexibility. Conversely, if a parent adopts a negative behaviour pattern within a consultation, it is likely that a child will also adopt this negativity. An extreme example is described by Runeson et al. (2002) who observed parents of 24 children aged 5 months to 18 years during admission to hospital with the aim of describing their degree of participation in decisions concerning their child's care.[15] These authors report that in some cases of low levels of child participation the parents showed no signs of supporting their child; they did not listen to the child's wishes, they did not question painful procedures in front of health professionals or demand a new approach or request alternative solutions.[15] One can see in this situation that it is likely that the child will 'withdraw' from taking part in the consultation and may even be exposed to unnecessary pain and distress.

Children learn through observing significant adults in their life.[30] Parents can facilitate child participation in consultations by using positive, active parental modelling. This method if adopted by parents will have a significant influence on whether children are involved in consultations within healthcare settings.[25]

GUIDANCE FOR PARENTS

Written guidance for parents within the emergency care setting regarding how to facilitate and support children during a consultation is sparse. Even within the wider literature there is an emphasis on tools for parents to test doctors on their ability to encourage child participation to assist in medical training rather than to provide a layperson's guide for parents.[31] Cunningham and Newton (2000) undertook work within paediatric neurology in the UK testing a question sheet to enable parents and children to get the information they want from consultations.[32] These authors addressed the need for a simple and effective intervention in the consultation which empowered parents to take control.[32] A further question sheet to guide parents to prepare for an active role in consultations is presented in the box entitled, 'A checklist for parents', which aims to maximise child participation (*see* p. 178). The checklist embodies the ethos of parental participation described in this chapter and adds other parent-centred ideas for consideration. It can be used by parents attending the emergency care environment or any healthcare setting.

CONCLUSIONS

The participation of children and young people in consultations rests heavily on the ability of the parent to facilitate and support the child. Current direct evidence which guides parents how to achieve such involvement is sparse within emergency care settings, which is contrary to national-level policy and the wider growing body of literature on parental and child participation. However, parents are encouraged to adopt active roles and proactive methods of preparation and parental modelling to achieve successful consultations from their own and their child's perspective. It is clear that development of high levels of child participation must also involve high levels of positive parental participation. Some techniques as discussed are extensions of everyday parenting techniques, therefore parents should not be fearful of what is involved in promoting child participation. Parental involvement is not a dichotomy of involved or not involved and indeed the parent needs to remain flexible reflecting the child's wishes and the clinical scenario presenting to the emergency department. However, opportunities for such child and parent participation in consultation in the emergency care environment are plentiful and should not be disregarded as inappropriate in this setting.

A checklist for parents

The guide consists of a list of 12 questions that you may wish to consider before, during and after the consultation. You as a parent will need to decide which questions are meaningful to you, your child and the situation. It is recommended that most of these are carefully considered before the consultation but it can also be used as a quick reminder during the consultation to help your child to feel fully involved or if time is limited.

1. To what level does your child want to participate? Choose one of the levels of participation described by Shier.[10,11]
2. What questions or issues does your child want to address in the consultation? Write them down or even better ask your child to write them down if they are old enough. If there is time, take a copy each.
3. Have you decided who will speak in which part of the consultation? For example, will your child answer questions about the symptoms and you as parent agree to a proposed management plan – aim to work as a team.
4. Are you and each adult coming with your child to the consultation keen to encourage them to take part fully in their consultation? Iron out any differences before the consultation.
5. Have you prepared your child so that they might get the best from the consultation? And, more importantly, agreed with them that the consultation will take place at all?
6. Have you decided how many parents or carers should go along with the child to the consultation?
7. Have you decided if other children such as brothers or sisters need or want to attend?
8. What should you take with you? Consider taking the following: a list of what is wrong with your child (e.g. a record of their last temperature), pen and paper (to help you remember what was decided), a list of your and your child's questions. No matter how tempting, do not take a sheaf of Internet print-outs, the health professionals will not have time to read them and they may not be accurate.
9. Have you thought how best you could 'model' how you want your child to behave in the consultation? If you think any particular issues will be difficult, it's worth thinking about how you will behave when these are addressed.
10. Are you aware of what NOT to do in the consultation?
    - Do not interrupt your child's responses to the health professional (evidence suggests that this causes the health professional to redirect their questions to the parent).
    - Do not answer questions on the child's behalf (although this can be a natural loving response from a parent it will stop your child from contributing).
    - Do not tell your child off for interrupting the discussion with their own questions.

- Do not tell your child to stay quiet while you speak to the health professional. This is a hard habit to break!
11. After the consultation, can you think of any further questions for next time or how they could be addressed in the meantime?
12. Allow your child to go back to normal activities (illness or injury permitting) but when will be a good time to ask how they thought it went and answer any questions they have?

REFERENCES

1 Intercollegiate Committee for Services for Children in Emergency Departments. *Services for Children in Emergency Departments*. London: Royal College of Paediatrics and Child Health; 2007.

2 Wissow LS, Roter D, Bauman LJ, *et al.* Patient–provider communication during the emergency department care of children with asthma. *Med Care*. 1998; **36**(10): 1439–50.

3 Alberti G. *Emergency Care Ten Years On: reforming emergency care*. London: Department of Health; 2007.

4 Bradley T, McCann B, Glasgow J, *et al.* Paediatric consultation patterns in general practice and the accident and emergency department. *Ulster Med J*. 1995; **64**(1): 51–7.

5 Hemingway P. Determining why parents with sick children attend Accident and Emergency and General Practice. University of Nottingham; PhD thesis 2004.

6 Child Health Support Group. *A Consultation on Emergency Care for Ill and Injured Children and Young People in Scotland*. Edinburgh: Scottish Executive; 2004.

7 Rise MB, Steinsbekk A. How do parents of child patients compare consultations with homeopaths and physicans? A qualitative study. *Patient Educ Couns*. 2009; **74**: 91–6.

8 Francis N, Wood F, Simpson S, *et al.* Developing an 'interactive' booklet on respiratory tract infections in children for use in primary care consultations. *Patient Educ Couns*. 2008; **73**: 286–93.

9 Goymour KL, Stephenson C, Goodenough B, *et al.* Evaluating the role of play therapy in the paediatric emergency department. *Aust Emerg Nurs J*. 2000; **3**(2): 10–12.

10 Shier H. Pathways to participation: openings, opportunities and obligations. *Child Soc*. 2001; **15**: 107–17.

11 Davies S, Thurston M. *Consulting with Children Under Five: a literature review. Executive summary. 1–21*. Chester: University of Chester; 2006.

12 Alderson P. *Young Children's Rights*. London: Jessica Kingsley Publishers; 2000.

13 Tates K, Meeuwesen L, Bensing J, *et al.* Joking or decision-making? Affective and instrumental behaviour in doctor–parent–child communication. *Psychol Health*. 2002; **17**(3): 281–95.

14 Rylance G. How do paediatricians communicate with children and parents? *Acta Pædiatr*. 2004; **93**(11): 1501–6.

15 Runeson I, Hallstrom I, Elander G, *et al.* Children's participation in the decision-making process during hospitalization: an observational study. *Nurs Ethics*. 2002; **9**: 583–98.

16 Wissow LS, Bar-Din Kimel M. Assessing provider–patient–parent communication in the pediatric emergency department. *Ambul Pediatr*. 2002; **2**(4 Suppl.): 323–9.

17 Harmsen H, Meeuwesen L, Wieringen J, *et al.* When cultures meet in general practice: intercultural differences between GPs and parents of child patients. *Patient Educ Couns.* 2003; **51**: 99–106.

18 Coyne I. Consultation with children in hospital: children, parents' and nurses' perspectives. *J Clin Nurs.* 2006; **15**: 61–71.

19 Young B, Dixon-Woods M, Windridge KC, *et al.* Managing communication with young people who have potentially life threatening chronic illness: qualitative study of patients and parents. *Brit Med J.* 2003; **326**: 305–10.

20 Alderson P, Sutcliffe K, Curtis K. Children as partners with adults in their medical care. *Arch Dis Child.* 2006; **91**: 300–3.

21 Jackson C, Cheater FM, Reid I. A systematic review of decision support needs of parents making child health decisions. *Health Expect.* 2008; **11**: 232–51.

22 Savage E, Callery P. Clinic consultations with children and parents on the dietary management of cystic fibrosis. *Soc Sci Med.* 2007; **64**: 363–74.

23 Gabe J, Olumide G, Bury M. 'It takes three to tango': a framework for understanding patient partnership in paediatric clinics. *Soc Sci Med.* 2004; **59**: 1071–9.

24 Hallstrom I, Elander G. Decision-making during hospitalization: parents' and children's involvement. *J Clin Nurs.* 2004; **13**: 367–75.

25 Coyne I. Children's participation in consultations and decision-making at health service level: a review of the literature. *Int J Nurs Stud.* 2008; **45**: 1682–9.

26 Jolley J. Commentary on Coyne I (2006). Consultation with children in hospital: children, parents' and nurses' perspectives. *J Clin Nurs.* 2006; **15**: 785–99.

27 Mathes E. Maslow's heirarchy of needs as a guide for living. *J Humanist Psychol.* 1981; **21**: 69–72.

28 Winskill R, Andrews D. Minimizing the 'ouch' – a strategy to minimize pain, fear and anxiety in children presenting to the emergency department. *Aust Emerg Nurs J.* 2008; **11**(4): 184–8.

29 Gerull FC, Rapee RM. Mother knows best: effects of maternal modelling on the acquisition of fear and avoidance behaviour in toddlers. *Behav Res Ther.* 2002; **40**: 279–87.

30 Mavor T. Like parent, like child: a health promoting hospital project. *Patient Educ Couns.* 2001; **45**: 261–4.

31 Crossley J, Eiser C, Davies HA. Children and their parents assessing the doctor–patient interaction: a rating system for doctor's communication skills. *Med Educ.* 2005; **39**: 820–8.

32 Cunningham C, Newton R. A question sheet to encourage written consultation questions. *Qual Health Care.* 2000; **9**: 42–6.

Index